'As a DMD Pathfinder, living with Duchenne, I t... this ... make a fantastic addition to the literature alrea... published. It's a thought provoking book that will give clinicians, teachers and parents an insight into all issues associated with the condition. Although they are aware of the physical effects of DMD, teachers and parents may not always realise that some children also have learning and behaviour problems. This book will support young people with DMD and their families to find solutions ahead of problems, so that they can transition into adulthood with the best support possible, and make the most of all opportunities.'

– Tyran Hawthorn, Trustee of DMD Pathfinders

'There is much to recommend this wide-ranging reference for the DMD community – from the importance of phonics mastery to job seeking. The most valuable advice from the contributors calls for: active listening, holding long-term expectations, individual goal setting and mindfulness in all things. Stakeholders will be bolstered to learn more and to expect local specialists and providers to approach problems with a solutions focus.'

– Deborah Robins, parent and Muscular Dystrophy Queensland Ambassador

'This truly is a go-to guide; written in such a clear format and with the breadth of important aspects of living with Duchenne. Following from Action Duchenne's learning and behavioural toolkit, this will prove an invaluable resource to the community and complements the forthcoming updated standard of care guidelines. Very positive and inspirational, a must-read for all.'

– Diana Ribeiro, Chief Executive Officer and Director of Research, Action Duchenne

'This inspirational book goes 'above and beyond' the journey of the physical and medical challenges associated with Duchenne Muscular Dystrophy (DMD). Case studies that will touch your soul but inspire your heart. Offering refreshing, crisp, deeper perspectives supporting parents, teachers and clinicians; to focus on the individual person and not just their condition on their road to adulthood.'

– Christopher Wilson, Deputy Head Teacher, Wilson Stuart School (Special Academy for young people with physical disabilities and complex medical needs)

'With medical interventions, boys with Duchenne are living into adult years. Traditionally, social and educational expectations have been lacking. This book will challenge your expectations as a parent or teacher. Encompassing neuro-developmental disorders associated with Duchenne, this book offers developmental recommendations for interventions, and empowers parents to successfully support boys into adulthood.'

– Michelle Pomeroy, Developmental Educator and mother of a boy with Duchenne

'Our son, Fraser, is 17 and has DMD and ASD. He also has specific learning difficulties associated with DMD. I am sure that both parents and professionals would benefit greatly from this book. Many professionals who worked with Fraser in his early years, especially in mainstream educational settings, would have gained much from it. DMD is a rare condition and add to that the complications of behavioural and learning difficulties and there are few who have the skills and/or the will to go beyond the standard interventions. If they had had access to straightforward information about the issues and guidance on how to address them many difficulties would have been avoided. The book is a "go to" source of information, inspiration and signposting and will encourage parents to be more creative and assertive in trying to ensure their children have good lives.'

– Julia Carr, parent to a teen with DMD and ASD, Gateshead

'This book is an accessible and actionable study looking at the lesser known barriers to learning and behaviour that young people with DMD experience. It guides teachers and parents to explore how starting early, self-determination, wellbeing and aspiration really matter, not just the focus on physical health. Essential reading for anyone involved in developing aspirations for young people with DMD.'

– Margaret Mulholland, Director of Development and Research, Swiss Cottage School Development and Research Centre

'This book is long overdue and will be a welcome resource for parents, caregivers, teachers and patients with Duchenne Muscular Dystrophy. It provides a compass with which to navigate the world of Duchenne Muscular Dystrophy, giving patients and caregivers the tools they need to manage the emotional, behavioural and learning challenges that sit alongside the physical realities of DMD. I found the chapter on talking to your children especially helpful, as I am very often asked by families when is the "right time" to tell their children. This books shows that although there is no right time, there are ways of addressing these unbelievably difficult conversations that will help. And there is lots else in the book to give parents the hope that their children can shoot for the stars and create as Dr Jon Hastie so movingly describes, a "fantastic life".'

– Emily Crossley, Co-Founder and Co-CEO,
Duchenne UK and Mum to Eli with DMD

'This book gives an excellent overview of DMD and provides a very valuable guide to the journey made for both parents and professionals. It has concise easy-to-read details on the complexities that come with DMD and practical tips. I particularly enjoyed reading about the inspirational adults with DMD and would highly recommend this book to all affected by Duchenne.'

– Claire Bosanquet, parent to two sons with DMD

'The practical guidance included in this book, with chapters on behaviour, EHC plans, transitioning to adulthood and work, will be invaluable to all parents, educators and health professionals supporting a young person with DMD. It's a must read which you will return to again and again.'

– Claire Binns, SENCO, Frederick Bremer School, Walthamstow

A Guide to Duchenne Muscular Dystrophy

of related interest

College for Students with Disabilities
We Do Belong
Edited by Pavan John Antony and Stephen M. Shore
ISBN 978 1 84905 732 5
eISBN 978 1 78450 101 3

Special Needs and Legal Entitlement, Second Edition
The Essential Guide to Getting out of the Maze
Melinda Nettleton and John Friel
ISBN 978 1 84905 706 6
eISBN 978 1 78450 230 0

The Parents' Guide to Specific Learning Difficulties
Information, Advice and Practical Tips
Veronica Bidwell
ISBN 978 1 78592 040 0
eISBN 978 1 78450 308 6

Specific Learning Difficulties – What Teachers Need to Know
Diana Hudson
Illustrated by Jon English
ISBN 978 1 84905 590 1
eISBN 978 1 78450 046 7

Defying Disability
The Lives and Legacies of Nine Disabled Leaders
Mary Wilkinson
ISBN 978 1 84310 415 5
eISBN 978 1 84642 083 2

A GUIDE TO DUCHENNE MUSCULAR DYSTROPHY

Information and Advice for Teachers and Parents

EDITED BY JANET HOSKIN

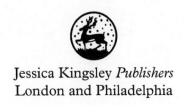

Jessica Kingsley *Publishers*
London and Philadelphia

First published in 2018
by Jessica Kingsley Publishers
73 Collier Street
London N1 9BE, UK
and
400 Market Street, Suite 400
Philadelphia, PA 19106, USA

www.jkp.com

Library of Congress Cataloging in Publication Data
Names: Hoskin, Janet, editor.
Title: A guide to Duchenne muscular dystrophy : information and advice for
   teachers and parents / edited by Janet Hoskin.
Description: London ; Philadelphia : Jessica Kingsley Publishers, 2018. |
   Includes bibliographical references and index.
Identifiers: LCCN 2017029942 | ISBN 9781785921650 (alk. paper)
Subjects: LCSH: Duchenne muscular dystrophy.
Classification: LCC RJ482.D78 G85 2018 | DDC 362.19892/748--dc23 LC record available at
https://lccn.loc.gov/2017029942

British Library Cataloguing in Publication Data
A CIP catalogue record for this book is available from the British Library

ISBN 978 1 78592 165 0
eISBN 978 1 78450 434 2

Printed and bound by CPI Group (UK) Ltd, Croydon, CR0 4YY

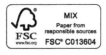

This book is dedicated to Saul, Mimi, Davy-Ray and Nick and to all the young people and adults with DMD and their families who I have been privileged to know over the past seventeen years, some of whom are no longer with us.

Contents

Introduction

DMD IN A NEW LANDSCAPE

Janet Hoskin

You are probably reading this book because you are a parent or teacher of a child with Duchenne Muscular Dystrophy (DMD); you may even have DMD yourself. This book aims to offer information and strategies that can help with the journey through school and beyond. It is not primarily about the physical or medical challenges associated with DMD, with just one chapter (Chapter 3) dedicated to exploring physical management of DMD. Rather, this book predominantly focuses on the lesser known barriers to learning and behaviour that many children and young people with DMD experience, and offers advice for parents, teachers and young people themselves on how to manage them. Above all, it is about supporting young people with DMD to get the life that they want.

You may well be aware that DMD is a rare genetic muscle wasting impairment that is caused by a fault on the dystrophin gene. This fault prevents a protein called dystrophin from being made. The protein dystrophin plays an important role in our muscle cells and without it the muscles of young people with DMD degenerate and grow progressively weaker. On average this means they lose the ability to walk around the age of 12 years (Bushby *et al.* 2010). Life expectancy is affected, and in 2007 the average was reported to be 27 years (Eagle *et al.* 2007). DMD predominantly affects boys because it is on the X-chromosome, but a very tiny number of girls are known to be affected.

A new landscape

In the early 1980s it was noted how schools might find it challenging teaching young people with DMD who would not survive into adulthood (Leibowitz and Dubowitz 1981). We are now living in a new landscape and we have to start with the premise that most children with DMD will grow up to be adults. Twenty years ago, young people died before they reached the age of 20, but with treatments such as cardiac management, steroids and most importantly night ventilation, men with DMD are living into their third and sometimes even fourth decades (Landfeldt et al. 2015).

Recently I was very fortunate to travel to Denmark where I met with adults with DMD living independently with support in their own homes. There are now more adults living with DMD in Denmark than children, and some live into their forties and fifties. I am not suggesting that there are not still too many of our young people whose lives are cut short, or that DMD is not a challenging and at times heart-breaking impairment to deal with. However, overwhelmingly we are seeing young people with DMD living into adulthood and this has important consequences for us as teachers and parents. It means we need to help our children prepare for life as an adult, rather than focus solely on them being happy in the here and now.

I am aware this book could be viewed as just adding more labels to children who already live with significant challenges. However, with DMD it is impossible to ignore what has been described as the 'impairment effects' and these are not just physical (Thomas 1999). Heightened risks of reading difficulties, social communication and behaviour differences have been established by a range of authors (Astrea et al. 2015; Billard et al. 1998; Hendriksen and Vles 2008; Hinton et al. 2004). In 2005, adults with DMD in Denmark reported that although they have a good quality of life, they regretted their lack of formal qualifications which can be important currency for entering the job market (Rahbek et al. 2005). Although of course not the only explanation, early targeted support in literacy and other lagging skills could help improve this situation for many young people with DMD.

The problem of low expectations

In Chapter 4, I talk about schools often feeling like they need 'permission' to challenge young people with DMD. Instead of putting in place what they would offer any other child presenting with similar learning challenges, teachers may hesitate because of the serious nature of the impairment. Often expectations can be low, particularly if a child, who already has a complex diagnosis, appears to struggle with communication or concentration. If children with DMD are given the support early, in most cases they will develop skills to read which will not only help them to access more opportunities as they live into adulthood, but reduce their risk of isolation. I have met too many young people who have had little or no expectations made of them academically. This has sometimes resulted in their transfer to specialist provision where they have not been entered for examinations, even though, with the appropriate support, many could have been successful. Of course, life isn't just about passing academic assessments and all children with DMD are different; for many children sitting formal examinations would not be appropriate. However, qualifications or training at whatever level, can at the very least make access to an interesting work-place easier and help us learn new skills.

Research in the UK on transition to adulthood in DMD has shown that even those adults who did not experience any difficulties at school have been affected by low expectations. Overwhelmingly adults with DMD have lived at home with their parents, have not had jobs and have very often been socially isolated (Abbott, Carpenter and Bushby 2012). There are many reasons for this, including attitudes in society that not only put barriers in the way of disabled people but serve to reduce their confidence and self-belief. However, as you will read in this book, with the appropriate support and high expectations young people with DMD can achieve employment, and live independently if this is what they aspire to. Employment does not have to be 'nine till five' Monday to Friday, or a daily journey into work. In England, the new Special Educational Needs and Disability (SEND) Reforms have introduced a focus on preparing for the world of work through initiatives such as supported internships and apprenticeships (DfE and DoH 2015). Some young people may choose to 'job carve', that is share a full time post with someone else, whereas others may prefer to be self-employed. However, what employment gives us, as well as the ability to pay the rent or mortgage, is the opportunity to meet a network of people who we can socialise with as well as do something we feel is meaningful and interesting.

How to use this book
Understanding the science

If you are a parent you may well have spent a lot of time and energy getting to grips with the science of DMD, particularly if your child has been included in any clinical trials. In **Chapter 1**, Kate Maresh and Francesco Muntoni will explain why DMD affects the brain as well as muscles. They will give an overview of the research about learning and behaviour differences in DMD, and why these occur. Through explaining the genetic roots of DMD we can understand why some young people may struggle more than others. There is still relatively little published data on DMD and the brain and the impact this can have on young people. Of course there is far more to us than our genes, and the rest of the book will look at ways that we, as parents and teachers, can support young people to have the best life possible as they become adults.

Understanding the key learning and behaviour challenges

Several of the chapters discuss the key barriers to learning that a young person with DMD may experience. **Chapter 2**, written by Veronica Hinton, uses four fictional case studies, to discuss strengths and difficulties that she has found young people with DMD experience through the considerable research she has undertaken. Of course all children are different, but Veronica has shown young people with DMD are at higher risk of specific difficulties that can impact on their learning, as well as likely to have strengths in particular areas. If you are in charge of Special Education in a school, or a psychologist assessing a young person with DMD, this chapter will help you understand some of the learning challenges and also the strengths that young people with DMD can experience. It will help you think about the type of assessments you might use, and how you might interpret some of the findings.

Chapter 3 is the only chapter in this book dedicated to the physical challenges facing those with DMD and how to manage them. Victoria Selby and Lianne Abbott, from Great Ormond Street Hospital, London, give advice on physiotherapy suitable for children with DMD and how as parents and teachers we can support this to happen. They discuss the various challenges facing young people with DMD at different ages, emphasising the importance of making exercise fun.

Chapter 4 may help those of you who have children who are younger and in primary or elementary schools. This chapter focuses on things to think about as your child begins his journey through school. I will share what established research tells us about younger children with DMD, and why we all need to understand that DMD is neuro-developmental as well as neuromuscular. In this way, we can appreciate some of the struggles children with DMD face. This chapter also underlines the central role we as parents and teachers can play in supporting them to develop knowledge and skills. I will also suggest some interventions that may help with early reading and learning at school and home and I will discuss the role of the teaching assistant.

Coping with difficult and challenging behaviour

Behaviour difficulties associated with DMD have only been acknowledged relatively recently. **Chapter 5** is written by James Poysky, who is a neuro-psychologist and practising child psychotherapist as well as a parent of a young person with DMD. James gives an overview of what research tells of behaviour risks, including externalising, internalising and social communication differences. Most helpfully he shares strategies that can be employed by parents and teachers to support young people who have confrontational or inflexible behaviour. James weaves his own personal and professional experience into this advice which is both humorous and extremely insightful. He helps us to see that traditional rewards and consequences often do not work and how we can best engage and support children to take responsibility for their actions.

Talking to children about DMD

In order to ensure that our children feel safe and confident, it is important to talk to them about DMD. **In Chapter 6** David Schonfeld tells us how important it is to make sure we do not avoid talking to children about DMD, but rather enable them to understand what it means in an age-appropriate way. Not speaking about it can create anxiety and lack of trust and uncertainty. As parents we are given this diagnosis, often with very little support, and often feel, through our own grief, that it is difficult to talk about it to our children. Sometimes waiting for the right moment just never seems to happen. David tells us that it's never too late to begin these conversations, and if we can start doing this now it can help our children to feel more in control of their lives.

Planning for now and a brighter future

We know that young people are living longer, but in order to get the life they want, adequate resources must be available. In **Chapter 7** Nick Catlin talks about getting the right plan in place for this. Although this chapter is primarily talking about the new Education Health and Care Plans that have been introduced in England, it provides key information to help you think about everything you need regardless of where you live. Very little in life can happen without a plan, particularly if you are living with a complex impairment. Most importantly, young people must now be consulted about what they want to do with their lives and this process must not be tokenistic. Although all children with DMD are unique and have different needs and dreams, most will need similar resources at various stages of their life, and making sure you have all this included in your plan is crucial. The new focus in the SEND Reforms on life outcomes rather than provision means that you must link everything you include in your plan to a particular outcome. Young people with Special Educational Needs in England can now ask for their plans to be maintained until the age of 25 years if they wish to continue in education.

Another impact of this new legislation is a chapter dedicated to Transition to Adulthood in the Special Needs and Disability Code of Practice (DfE and DoH 2015). All children in England with Special Educational Needs between the ages of 14 and 19 years should now be asked in their annual reviews what they hope to do in the future in the areas of employment, housing, developing and maintaining friendships and their health. In **Chapter 8**, myself and Celine Barry share the lessons we have learned from running the lottery-funded Transition to Adulthood project 'Takin' Charge' which worked with over 80 young people with DMD who were between the ages of 14 and 19 years and their families. This project supported young people with DMD to think seriously about their future. As well as developing a range of creative projects we brought together professionals from supported employment and housing organisations and those experienced in running programmes on sexual health. Most of all we benefited from the input of a small group of adults with DMD who loyally supported us as a steering committee for the five years of the project.

Hearing from men with DMD

Two members of the Takin' Charge steering committee went on to establish the first organisation led by adults with DMD. **Chapter 9,** written by DMD Pathfinders founders Dr Jon Hastie and Mark Chapman, who are 36 and 47 years old respectively, gives an overview of life with DMD as adults who were not expected to be here. Among other things Jon tells us about his journey from school to university and ultimately to employment. Mark speaks about going to school and college away from home and living independently as an adult. He also shares his experience of having a tracheostomy at the age of 24.

Being a parent and teacher

When our children are diagnosed with DMD it is life changing. Initially we tend to focus on the physical aspects of the impairment, as these appear the most shocking. In fact, through our grief and trauma I don't think there is any room to consider anything else. We all react to the diagnosis in different ways – some of us start running marathons, some of us set up foundations or charities or start raising money for existing ones, others make it their mission to have the best family life ever. Whatever we do, it's important that we are surrounded by enough friends or family to support us and with whom we are able to talk about how we feel and how we are coping.

Initially you may feel like you don't want to meet other families affected by DMD, but engaging with the DMD community can be helpful and reassuring and is often a way of finding out about research as well as how to access necessary support and resources. Families affected by DMD are incredibly rich in knowledge and I would recommend either making local connections or attending events that are organised by user-led groups. Sometimes it can be lonely and, like other families with disabled children, you are made to feel 'different' by prevailing attitudes in society. Similarly, I have met teachers who have expressed the need to meet other professionals working with children with such a rare impairment. Opportunities for meeting up with other teachers or educators on training days or conferences can often be the key that opens a new and more effective way of working.

When we set up Parent Project UK (now Action Duchenne) in 2001, like many parents of children who are newly diagnosed with medical impairments, our sole aim was to find a cure. At that time, life expectancy was reported as being 19 years, and even though we were told at diagnosis about ventilation and steroid regimes, it was impossible to feel anything positive. Like parents before and after us, we felt broken and desperate and the only thing we could hold onto was the hope for a cure.

Over the next few years, as we built the charity and met other families, we began to realise that many parents were struggling on a daily basis with the demands of bringing up a child with DMD, even before they showed any signs of physical deterioration. At our annual conferences parents were reporting how their children were struggling to read, or behave in school, others had been advised that their children could not cope in a mainstream setting and needed to move to specialist provision. Often poor parenting was seen as the cause of these issues – our inability not to 'spoil' our children who had such a serious prognosis; other specialists advised that our children were not adjusting to having such a debilitating impairment and were 'playing up' because of it.

I am very confident that this book will serve to help you if you are a parent or teacher dealing with these issues right now and offer some insight and strategies. I also hope that it will encourage you to have the highest expectations for young people with DMD so that they are able to follow their dreams, whatever they may be, as they grow into adulthood. The last seven years of austerity in the UK have made it a particularly challenging time to be disabled, but as this book will advise, with a comprehensive plan, adequate resources, support from each other and a lot of grit and determination who knows what is possible?

Chapter One

WHY SOME CHILDREN WITH DMD HAVE LEARNING AND BEHAVIOUR DIFFICULTIES

Kate Maresh and Francesco Muntoni

As all parents and teachers know, every child is different. And this is just as true for a child with Duchenne Muscular Dystrophy (DMD) as it is for a child without the condition. However, parents, teachers and clinicians would all agree that there are certain patterns of learning and behaviour differences in some children with DMD compared to children without the condition. For example, young boys with DMD often learn to speak later than boys in the general population, and are more likely experience a range of different learning and behaviour difficulties (Cyrulnik *et al.* 2007; Snow, Anderson and Jakobson 2013). As these features are not observed in other conditions that equally affect motor abilities, this suggests that DMD affects the brain as well as the muscles.

Knowing how the brain can be affected in DMD is important. While learning and behaviour differences do not occur in every child with DMD, recognising that they are more common may help specific strengths and difficulties to be identified at an early age. This will help parents, teachers and health care professionals to make early interventions so every child with DMD can reach their full intellectual potential and reduce the chance of mental health problems.

In this chapter, we will start with an overview of some of the differences that can occur in learning and behaviour in DMD boys, on which subject more detail will also be provided in Chapter 2. We will then explain what is known about the science behind these differences between different DMD boys. This will focus on how the different changes in the genetic code can change how the brain functions, affecting some children severely while sparing others. Finally, we will look at how this information may be used in the future in a way that can support boys and young men with the condition.

What are the learning and behaviour differences?

It is important to remember that many boys with DMD do not have differences in learning and behaviour compared to children without the condition. However, in some boys with DMD their learning and behaviour can be affected, at times quite significantly. There are also many highly intelligent young people with DMD who now progress well through school and into further study or work, especially now that there are improved opportunities for people with physical disabilities.

From the evidence to date, the effects of DMD on the brain seem to be separate from the effects on muscle. That is, while the muscle condition gradually worsens over time, there is no evidence that brain function worsens (Emery, Muntoni and Quinlivan 2015). Indeed, some aspects such as language difficulties may improve with time, as described below. In addition, the severity of the muscle condition does not relate to the degree of brain-related impairment.

Learning differences

In the past, the scientific research into learning difficulties in DMD has mainly focused on intellectual disability, usually recording the Intelligence Quotient (IQ) as this is a standardised measure. According to papers published between 1960 and 2016 the average IQ of boys with DMD was 85, compared to a general population average of 100. This included a large study which combined information from many papers and included over 1200 boys (Cotton, Voudoris and Greenwood 2001). This study also showed that intellectual disability (IQ <70) occurs in about a third of boys with DMD compared to 1–3 per cent in the general population (McKenzie *et al.* 2016).

However, although IQ tests are commonly used, there are problems with using a single IQ score as a way of assessing intellectual function. An IQ score alone does not give a full picture of an individual's learning ability or disability, particularly if there are large differences in the scores between different sections of the test. Looking at these sub-test scores can give us a better picture of the specific strengths and weaknesses that an individual may have. For example, common areas of strength in DMD children include memory for fact-based knowledge, vocabulary and spatial awareness, whereas difficulties can occur with the understanding of words and language, attention and memory, particularly the 'working memory' required for processing language, known as verbal working memory (Hinton *et al.* 2001). Indeed, some of the difficulties boys face when they are younger may be due to understanding and processing language, with older boys scoring more highly in these sections of the intelligence tests than younger boys (Cyrulnik *et al.* 2007).

Other indications that language is particularly affected include a delay in learning to speak in 60–70 per cent of young boys (Parsons, Clarke and Bradley 2004; Smith *et al.*1989). Reading difficulties in school age children occur in 40–70 per cent of boys, including a reading age two years behind that of the boys' peers, despite normal scores on the 'performance' part of the IQ tests (which include reasoning and visuo-spatial function) (Astrea *et al.* 2015; Billard *et al.* 1992; Billard *et al.* 1998).

Other aspects of learning that may be affected in DMD include difficulties with mathematics and writing, as well as problems with what is known as 'executive function' (Donders and Taneja 2009). Executive function is a way of controlling tasks that are performed by other parts of the brain to optimise performance. Problems in this system can lead to difficulties with planning, and with being flexible in adapting to different tasks and focusing attention.

Behavioural and other brain-related differences

Several other brain-related co-morbidities occur more often in DMD than in the general population. These include behavioural problems, attention deficit hyperactivity disorder, anxiety, depression, autism spectrum disorder, obsessive compulsive disorder and epilepsy (Hendriksen *et al.* 2015; Ricotti *et al.* 2016b; Snow *et al.* 2013). While many children may occasionally show behavioural disturbance, such as aggression or disruptiveness, these behaviours can become a problem when they start to interfere with daily life.

Attention deficit hyperactivity disorder (ADHD) is a condition in which children show inattention, hyperactivity and impulsivity, although not necessarily all three. In autism spectrum disorder (ASD) there are problems with social interaction and communication, as well as restricted interests and rigid or repetitive behaviours. Anxiety, such as a feeling of unease, worry or fear, is a common reaction to change or life stresses in children. But if it affects their thoughts and behaviour on a daily basis it can become a problem. Anxiety can be generalised or more specific, such as social phobia or obsessive compulsive disorder (OCD). In OCD an obsessive thought repeatedly enters your mind and leads to unpleasant feelings and anxiety, for example that your hands are dirty. A compulsive behaviour is then done to try to temporarily relieve the anxiety; for example, repeatedly washing your hands. Depression is a condition of persistent low mood, and can include symptoms such as unhappiness, irritability and unexplained tearfulness. Epilepsy is a condition that affects the brain and causes repeated fits, known as seizures.

There has been less research into these other conditions in DMD. However, we have reviewed all the relevant research studies over the past few decades to assess how commonly these conditions occur in DMD compared to children in the general population (Maresh and Muntoni, 2017). These findings are presented in in Table 1.1.

Some of these differences are striking, however it is worth bearing in mind several things when considering such numbers. First, while this shows that on average one out of five boys with DMD (20 per cent) will have a diagnosis of ADHD, four out of five boys with DMD will not. Also in the general population, approximately one in 10–20 boys (5–10 per cent) are said to have ADHD.

Second, the findings vary between studies so these are only estimates of how common these conditions are in DMD. For example, in one study that looked at ADHD in children with DMD, over half of all the children in the study had this diagnosis, whereas in another study only 7.5 per cent (approximately 1 in 13) children had this diagnosis (Humbertclaude et al. 2013; Pane et al. 2012). Therefore, to help to make sense of these figures we can get an idea how accurate the estimates are by looking at the 'confidence interval', which is the range of values that we would expect the true result to be within. In statistics we usually use a '95 per cent confidence interval', which tells us that we are 95 per cent confident that the estimate is within this range. The 95 per cent confidence intervals are shown in brackets below the main percentage figure in Table 1.1. Taking the example of ADHD again, we estimate that 20 per cent of boys with DMD also have ADHD, but we expect that the true estimate will be 20 per cent +/- 4.5 per cent, i.e. somewhere between 15.5 per cent and 24.5 per cent. This is still higher than the rate in the normal population so it is likely to be a fairly accurate reflection of how common ADHD is in DMD. The bigger the number of subjects studied, the more accurate the estimate will be, and, conversely, when there are fewer subjects included in a study the results are likely to be less accurate. For example, while the rate of epilepsy in DMD is found to be higher than in the general population (5 per cent vs. 0.5 per cent in the general population), we cannot be very confident of this as the confidence interval suggests that the true value may lie anywhere between -3.5 per cent and 13.5 per cent, and it is not possible to have a rate less than zero. Therefore this is an inaccurate estimate. From what we know, it is likely that epilepsy is more common in DMD, but, because of the small numbers investigated to date, the figures are inaccurate.

Table 1.1 Percentage of DMD boys and children in the general population with brain-related conditions

	Speech delay	Behavioural problems	Attention deficit hyperactivity disorder	Anxiety/ depression	Autism spectrum disorder	Obsessive compulsive disorder	Epilepsy
DMD	60–70% [1,2]	26% (+/- 6%) [3]	20% (+/- 4.5%) [3,6,7,8,9]	19% (+/- 5.5%) [3,6,9]	8% (+/- 6.5%) [6,7, 9,13,14, 15]	5% (+/- 9.5%) [6,7]	5% (+/- 8.5%) [18,19,20]
General population	6% [2]	5% [4,5]	3–9% [5,10,11]	2–3% [5,11,12]	1% [5,16,17]	2% [11]	0.5% [21]

Percentage figures in bold show estimates of the prevalence of different brain-related conditions in DMD in the first row and the general population in the second row. Figures in brackets give the 95 per cent confidence interval for these estimates in DMD: i.e. we are 95 per cent confident that the true figure lies within this range. Original source data references given below.

[1] *Parsons, Clarke and Bradley (2004);* [2] *Smith et al. (1989);* [3] *Caspers-Conway et al. (2015);* [4] *Brauner and Stephens (2006);* [5] *Green et al. (2005);* [6] *Banihani et al. (2015);* [7] *Hendriksen and Vles (2008);* [8] *Pane et al. (2012);* [9] *Ricotti et al. (2016b);* [10] *Blackburn and Spencer (2012);* [11] *Costello et al. (2003);* [12] *Cartwright-Hatton, McNicol and Doubleday (2006);* [13] *Darke et al. (2006);* [14] *Hinton et al. (2009);* [15] *Wu et al. (2005);* [16] *Fombonne (2003);* [17] *Van Naarden Braun et al. (2015);* [18] *Etemadifar and Molaei (2004);* [19] *Goodwin, Muntoni and Dubowitz (1997);* [20] *Pane et al. (2013);* [21] *Cowan (2002).*

As well as a small sample size, other reasons for inaccuracies in estimating how common these conditions are include: different ways of defining and testing for the conditions in different studies; differences within groups of children with DMD depending on their mutation in the DMD gene and age; a bias in the published results, or full data results not being published.

In summary, these figures can give us an indication of how common these conditions are based on research studies to date, however larger, more standardised studies are needed so that we can understand these relationships more clearly. Also, while these figures may be useful when considering a group of people as a whole, they are not always helpful when thinking about an individual. The bottom line is that while many children with DMD will not have these problems, a child with DMD is more likely to be affected than a child without DMD. This is important for parents, caregivers, teachers and clinicians to bear in mind so that if such problems are detected appropriate interventions can be put in place at an early age. It is well established that early intensive behavioural intervention has benefits in children with autism spectrum disorders, including increased IQ, and improved behaviour and adaptive skills. There is evidence that similar early intervention is also effective in children with learning and behaviour difficulties due to other causes, and has positive effects on parents, such as improved engagement and confidence (Eldevik *et al.* 2010; Guralnick 2016).

Overlapping brain-related disorders

It is well known that in the general population there can be an overlap of brain-related developmental disorders in a child, which include behavioural, emotional and cognitive disorders. For example, children with epilepsy and autism are more likely to have intellectual disability and ADHD, and up to half of children with ADHD will have co-occurring reading disability (Kaplan *et al.* 2001).

As Figure 1.1 shows, the same pattern can be seen in DMD. If a child has one brain-related disorder they are more likely to have another, demonstrating the overlap of different symptoms. These results come from a recent study which assessed 87 boys with DMD for intellectual disability, autism spectrum disorder, ADHD and emotional behavioural problems (which included anxiety, depression, aggression and hyperactivity). The researchers found that over a third of the boys had none of these problems (37 per cent), about a quarter (26 per cent) had one brain-related condition, and the remaining 37 per cent had two or more of these conditions (Ricotti *et al.* 2016b).

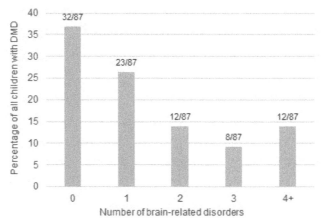

Figure 1.1 Bars show the number of overlapping brain-related disorders affecting boys with DMD. The vertical axis shows the percentage of boys in each category. Data labels show the number of boys in each category out of a total of 87.
(Data reproduced with permission from Ricotti et al. 2016b)

It is still not entirely clear why there is an additional association with DMD; however, the approach to supporting a child with DMD who also has several overlapping brain-related symptoms should be no different from a child without DMD.

Why does DMD affect the brain?

In the past, intellectual disability in DMD was thought to be caused by the physical disability reducing a child's educational opportunity. However, research studies have compared children with DMD to children with other diseases that cause a similar level of physical disability and found that children with DMD have more learning and behaviour challenges than children with other physical disabilities (Billard *et al.* 1992; Billard *et al.* 1998; Lorusso *et al.* 2013).

It is possible that a child might have learning difficulties unrelated to DMD, for example due to another cause of inherited learning disability. However, research has looked at the siblings of children with DMD and has shown that this is not the case. A boy with DMD is more likely to have learning and behaviour problems compared to an unaffected sibling (Hinton *et al.* 2000). This suggests that the differences in brain function are related to DMD rather than occurring by chance.

Laboratory studies in animals and people without DMD have shown that dystrophin is produced in specific areas of the brain (see Figure 1.7, p.32) (Lidov 1996; Sekiguchi *et al.* 2009). The brain-related problems in DMD are thought to be caused directly by the loss of the protein dystrophin in these brain regions. Dystrophin appears to have a major role in the transmission of nerve signals at certain types of nerve junctions in the brain (Perronnet and Vaillend 2010).

The nature of the genetic change in a person with DMD can, in some cases, also influence the degree to which the brain is affected (Muntoni, Torelli and Ferlini 2003). We will discuss below how these genetic differences can affect the brain function in DMD. But first it may be helpful to have an overview of some of the concepts in the genetics of DMD.

Genetics in DMD

The building blocks of life

Our bodies are made up of cells. Most cells contain a nucleus which is where our genes are stored. Genes are like instructions for health, growth and development of the human body. They are arranged on thread-like structures called chromosomes (see Figure 1.2). If a chromosome were a string of beads, then the genes are the beads on the string. Genes and chromosomes are made up of the same thing, which is a chemical called DNA. Every gene contains the instructions to make a different protein, and proteins are the building blocks of the body.

Humans have 23 pairs of chromosomes, of which one pair determines if we are male or female. These are called the X- or Y-chromosomes. Women have two X-chromosomes, whilst men have one X-chromosome and one Y-chromosome. A female inherits one X-chromosome from each parent, and a male inherits his X-chromosome from his mother and his Y-chromosome from his father. These 46 chromosomes are present in all the cells of the body and contain the genetic information required to make up a person.

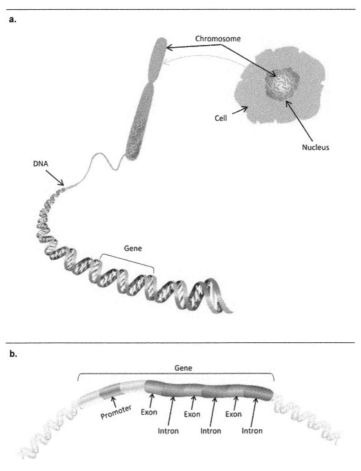

Figure 1.2 a) The structure of DNA and chromosomes. b) The structure of a gene.
(Adapted from the NHS HEE Genomics Education Programme)

Every gene is divided into sections called 'exons' and 'introns'. Exons contain the important genetic code which provides the instructions for making a protein. Introns are the sections of code in between the exons. The gene for DMD (called dystrophin) is one of the largest in humans and has 79 exons. This gene is the instruction to make a protein, which is also called dystrophin. Dystrophin is a very large protein which works in the muscles of the body (limbs, chest and heart) to stabilise muscle fibres and protect them from damage.

Mutations

Changes can occur in the genetic code. These are called 'mutations'. These can be passed down through the family or can be a new change in a child's genes. A mutation can change the way the protein is made and can have different effects. If a mutation does not change how the protein works then there will be no effect. However, sometimes a mutation may mean that a protein is changed or it cannot be produced at all. The effect of this depends on what that protein would normally do in the body, and can be either positive or negative.

Every person has two copies of each gene, one inherited from each parent, except in the case of the sex chromosomes (X and Y). This means that if there is a mutation in one gene, sometimes the other gene can compensate for it. But for genes on the X-chromosome the situation is different. Because of the way that it is inherited, a boy only has one copy of the X-chromosome whereas a girl has two.

The DMD gene is on the X-chromosome. If a girl has a mistake in the genetic code within the gene, then the copy of the DMD gene on the other X-chromosome can usually compensate. Therefore, a girl with the mutation may have no problems or only be mildly affected (although there are exceptions). If there is a mistake in the DMD gene on the boy's only X-chromosome, there is no 'back-up' copy so the protein production will be affected. This is why usually only boys are affected by DMD.

A mutation in the DMD gene can either stop the production of dystrophin almost completely or can lead to an altered protein being produced, which is not as effective as normal dystrophin. DMD is caused by a loss of almost all dystrophin. This means that the muscle fibres are not protected and they gradually become damaged and scarred. When an altered, less effective version of dystrophin is produced, muscle damage occurs more gradually and this leads to the milder condition Becker muscular dystrophy (BMD).

As DMD is a genetic condition, it can affect more than one member of the family. If you have any questions about the chance of other family members having DMD or having a child with DMD you can ask your doctor to refer you to your local genetics service to discuss this. This is called Genetic Counselling.

Different types of dystrophin

The dystrophin gene works in different ways in different parts of the body and the gene can create slightly different forms of dystrophin protein. These different forms are called 'isoforms'. The instructions to tell cells which isoforms to create are contained in the introns and in DNA code at the beginning and end of the gene, called 'promoters' (Muntoni *et al.* 2003).

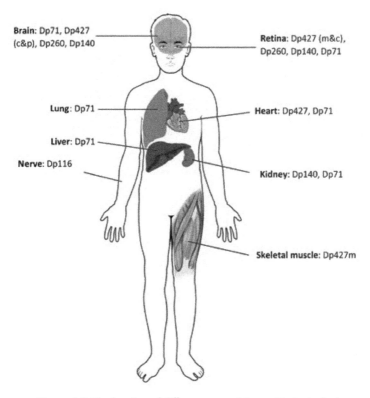

Brain: Dp71, Dp427 (c&p), Dp260, Dp140

Retina: Dp427 (m&c), Dp260, Dp140, Dp71

Lung: Dp71

Heart: Dp427, Dp71

Liver: Dp71

Nerve: Dp116

Kidney: Dp140, Dp71

Skeletal muscle: Dp427m

Figure 1.3 The location of different types of dystrophin in the body.
(Adapted from https://opentextbc.ca/anatomyandphysiology)

The isoforms are given a number which refers to their size, which is measured in kiloDaltons (a measure of the molecular size). The largest full-length dystrophin, found in muscle, is called Dp427m ('m' is for muscle). Two other proteins of the same size can also be produced in the brain, called Dp427c ('c' is for cortex – the outer layer of the brain) and Dp427p ('p' is for Purkinje – a type of cell in the part of the brain called the cerebellum) (Aartsma-Rus *et al.* 2006).

Smaller isoforms of dystrophin are produced in other organs of the body, including the brain, the eye, nerves, kidneys and liver (Figures 1.3 and 1.4). The smallest isoform, Dp71, is found in many different organs but it is the main type of dystrophin found in the brain.

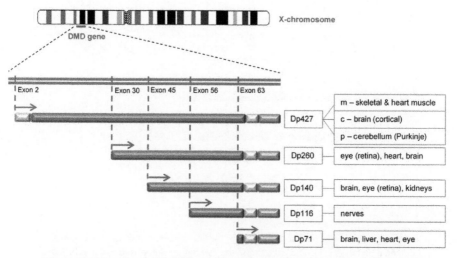

Figure 1.4 Diagram of the DMD gene, the different dystrophin protein isoforms and where they are found in the body. Dotted lines indicate where the 'reading' of the gene begins, in order to produce different isoforms of dystrophin. Arrows indicate the direction that the gene is 'read' in to produce the isoforms.

Most of our understanding of the dystrophin gene and isoforms comes from studies of dystrophin in animal models of DMD, such as mice. However, as the gene for dystrophin is very similar across animal species the findings can be to some extent extrapolated to DMD in humans.

We will discuss more about what is known about the role of dystrophin in the brain later in the chapter. But first we will consider how different genetic mutations may lead to differences in the brain.

The effects of the mutation site

In DMD the location of the mutation in the dystrophin gene determines which of these smaller proteins are kept or lost. Figure 1.5 shows that if the mutation is near the start of the gene (closer to exon 1), the largest protein (Dp427) will be lost but the smaller isoforms can still be made in their respective organs. However, if the mutation is towards the end of the gene then all or nearly all of the smaller forms will also be lost.

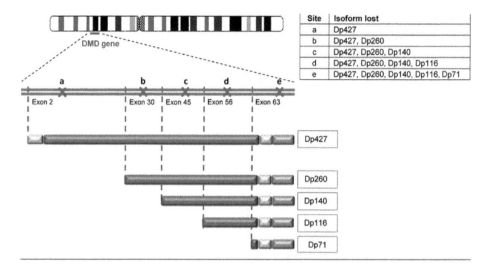

Figure 1.5 DMD gene and dystrophin isoforms. 'x' markers indicate examples of potential mutation sites. The table shows the dystrophin isoforms that would be lost because of mutations at each site.

The most important smaller isoforms with regards to learning differences are Dp71 and Dp140. In general, when the mutation is towards the end of the gene, i.e. when there is loss of the Dp140 and Dp71 isoforms, there are more likely to be learning differences than if the mutation is closer to the start of the gene, and when all isoforms are lost the consequences for brain function are typically more severe (Taylor *et al.* 2010). This is shown on the chart in Figure 1.6. There is a cumulative effect: for each additional isoform lost for mutations towards the end of the gene, there is an increased chance of learning difficulties, and these are likely to be more severe. For example in a recent review of the literature, boys with mutations at the end of the gene (equivalent to point 'e' on Figure 1.5) had an average IQ of 70, compared to boys with mutations near the start (point 'a') with an average IQ of 93 (Maresh and Muntoni, 2017).

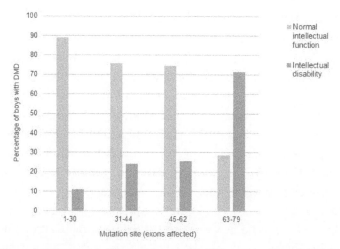

Figure 1.6 Percentage of boys with normal intellect and intellectual disability depending on their mutation site, shown by the exons affected and the types of dystrophin isoform lost.

There are fewer studies that relate other brain-related problems to the site of DMD gene mutations, so we do not have the clear correlation between genetics and these symptoms that we do for intellectual impairment. However, as a general rule boys with mutations towards the end of the gene tend to have more profound difficulties, which means they need more support with their learning (Ricotti *et al.* 2016b).

Genetics and the brain in DMD: Summary

We have now established that different mutations in the DMD gene can affect the types of dystrophin, or isoforms, that are produced in the brain. All boys with DMD are at increased risk of having learning and behaviour difficulties, but for those with mutations which cause many, or all, of the brain isoforms to be lost (including Dp140 and Dp71), there is a particularly increased risk of having learning difficulties. We also know that the smallest isoform of dystrophin, Dp71, is the main type of dystrophin found in the brain. So, the big question is: what do these dystrophin isoforms normally do in the brain? This is a subject that is still open to much scientific investigation; however, we will review what is currently known in the next section.

The function of dystrophin in the brain

There are two main theories of what dystrophin might do in the brain. The first possibility is that it is important in development of the brain, in which case any differences would be likely to be permanent. The second possibility is that it provides an ongoing role in brain function throughout life (Anderson, Head and Morley 2012; Chaussenot *et al.* 2015; Waite, Brown and Blake 2012). It is unlikely that treatment could improve a permanent change that was made when the brain was developing. However, if dystrophin has an ongoing role in the brain then it may be possible to improve the brain function by restoring the missing dystrophin proteins. These two theories are not necessarily mutually exclusive, and as we will see it is likely that dystrophin acts in both these ways.

Dystrophin and brain structure

Dystrophin is mainly found in certain areas of the brain, for example in parts of the outer layer of the brain, called the cortex, in small structures deep inside the brain, called the hippocampus and amygdala, and in the cerebellum, which is a structure at the back of the brain (see Figure 1.7) (Lidov 1996; Sekiguchi *et al.* 2009). These brain structures are highly interconnected with other areas of the brain, so it can be difficult to attribute all the features of a condition to particular brain areas. However, there are some associations that do seem relevant to the brain-related aspects of DMD, and may help us to understand what happens when dystrophin is lost.

The following is an overview of several areas of the brain that contain dystrophin and some of their functions which may be affected if dystrophin is lost. Dystrophin is produced in all areas of the cerebral cortex; however, an area towards the front of the brain called the prefrontal cortex seems to be particularly affected in DMD (Suzuki *et al.* 2017; Xu *et al.* 2015). The prefrontal cortex has connections to many parts of the brain; however, its functions include learning, memory and executive function (Groenewegen and Uylings 2000). The lateral, or outer, parts of cerebellum that connect to the cortex, are thought to be involved in certain aspects of cognition, such as verbal working memory and skill learning (Buckner 2013). The hippocampus is also involved in memory and the learning of facts, while the amygdala is involved in the processing of fear and emotion, and connects with the hippocampus for emotional learning (Bechara, Damasio and Damasio 2003; Le Doux 2003; McDonald and Mott 2017). The hippocampus is also an important structure in some types of epilepsy, and the cerebellum also may have a role in epilepsy (Hendriksen *et al.* 2016). There is still much that is unknown about how these areas and their connections are affected in DMD; however, as laboratory and brain imaging techniques advance our understanding will improve.

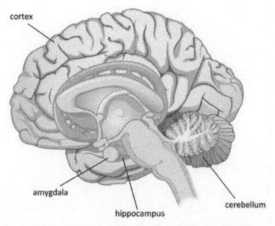

Figure 1.7 The areas of the brain in which dystrophin is produced.
(Adapted with permission from OpenStax Psychology)

Early studies of the brain did not show any obvious differences in the brain structure between children with DMD and those without DMD (Dubowitz and Crome 1969); however, using different brain scanning techniques, more recent studies have shown some subtle differences in both mice and humans with DMD (Goodnough *et al.* 2014; Lee *et al.* 2002). For example, a recent study showed that DMD children have a slightly smaller sized brain than children without DMD, although this difference was clearest in those children who had lost the Dp140 dystrophin isoform (Doorenweerd *et al.* 2014). However, there was no definite link between intellectual function and brain size, i.e. people with bigger brains did not necessarily have higher scores on IQ and other tests. Therefore, even if there is a small difference in brain size this does not necessarily affect how the brain works.

The Dp140 dystrophin isoform is present in the brain before birth, during brain development. Dp71 is also present before birth, and may help in the development of the protective barrier between the brain and the rest of the body, known as the blood-brain barrier (Nico *et al.* 2005). It has been suggested that lacking Dp140 and Dp71 alters the way the brain matures in the developing baby and this leads to a smaller brain size (Doorenweerd *et al.* 2014). So, dystrophin is likely to be important in the development of the brain before birth, but the smaller isoforms may have a bigger role than the full-length protein.

Dystrophin and brain function

The evidence for how dystrophin might work in the brain has come from two approaches. The first approach has been to study brain cells in the laboratory and see what happens when dystrophin is and is not present. The second approach has been to use gene therapy to restore dystrophin in experimental animals with DMD and to compare their behaviour with untreated animals.

Dystrophin in the cells of the brain

In muscle cells the full-length Dp427 protein forms a structural support in muscles. It stabilises muscle cells by linking the muscle fibres to other structural tissue in the muscle and connects with many other important proteins (Emery *et al.* 2015).

Dp427 dystrophin also appears to interact with other proteins in the nerve cells of the brain. These specialised proteins are called 'receptors' and are fixed to the surface of nerve cells. The receptors receive signals from other nerve cells via chemical messengers that move from one nerve cell to another at nerve endings, known as synapses. This is the way that signals are transmitted between nerves both in the brain and the rest of the body. Dystrophin may help to provide structural support for receptors at the end of the nerves and ensure that the receptors are in the correct place for the most effective signal transmission. If the receptors are not working properly then the signalling between nerve cells in the brain may be affected (Perronnet and Vaillend 2010).

Evidence from humans that disrupted nerve cell signalling is a part of DMD may be suggested by the fact that there is a higher chance of having epilepsy associated with DMD (see Table 1.1; Hendriksen *et al.* 2015). Seizures (fits) in epilepsy can occur when signalling goes wrong in the brain.

As mentioned above, the smallest dystrophin protein, Dp71, may also provide structural support within the reinforced lining of the blood vessels around the brain, known as the blood-brain barrier (Nico *et al.* 2005). The blood-brain barrier is made up of tightly connected cells that control the movement of substances into the brain from the bloodstream. Dp71 also interacts with proteins that allow water and other substances into and out of nerve cells in the brain (Perronnet and Vaillend 2010). If these carefully balanced systems are disturbed, we would predict that it would also disrupt how well the nerve cells of the brain can work.

Restoring dystrophin in the brain

Exon-skipping treatments are a recent development in the emerging therapies for DMD (Niks and Aartsma-Rus 2017). Exon-skipping therapy is a treatment that creates an almost full-length dystrophin protein that cannot normally be made in a mouse or human with DMD. The drug used is called an 'antisense oligonucleotide'. This is a small chemical that works like a patch by sticking to an area of DNA near the mutation in the DMD gene. This allows the faulty part of the gene to be skipped over, and an almost full-length protein is produced, with a part missing in the middle. Because the beginning and the end sections of the protein are present it can still interact with the other proteins that it needs to, and therefore still can have some useful function, although it is not as effective as the normal full-length protein.

Results from mice with DMD and early clinical trials in humans have shown that this modified dystrophin is effective in the muscles. The exon-skipping therapies currently in use in humans are not able to target the brain as they cannot cross the blood-brain barrier. Therefore, we do not know if they would be effective in the human brain.

However, mice with DMD have been treated with different exon-skipping drugs that can reach brain cells. Without treatment, these mice show several behaviours that we can compare to similar problems in humans. These include altered social behaviour and an exaggerated response to fear. All mice 'freeze' when they feel threatened, but in mice with DMD this response lasts for much longer than normal. When exon-skipping therapy was given to young mice, the abnormal freezing response was completely restored to normal after a few weeks of treatment (Goyenvalle *et al.* 2015; Sekiguchi *et al.* 2009). Exon-skipping therapy in these mice can also restore receptor proteins in nerve cells back to their correct location, which would be expected to improve nerve signalling (Vaillend *et al.* 2010).

Dystrophin in the eye

The nerve cell layer at the back of the eye is called the retina. The nerve cells in the retina detect light signals and transmit them via nerve pathways to the brain. Although the eye is not within the brain itself, as it is so closely connected it is a useful window into the brain.

The retina contains several types of dystrophin, as we saw earlier in Figures 1.3 and 1.4. A loss of dystrophin, particularly the smallest Dp71 dystrophin, can affect nerve signalling in the retina. These electrical signals can be recorded at the surface of the eye, and can therefore provide a non-invasive way of assessing nerve cell signalling (Ricotti *et al.* 2016a).

Although we can pick up small electrical changes in signalling in some children with DMD, this does not appear to have any effect on their vision. However, this observation may be very useful as a way of picking up changes due to dystrophin within the brain and the eye, which may become more relevant in the future if new drug therapies are targeted to the brain in DMD. Researchers have already tested this in mice with DMD. In a recent study, mice with DMD were treated with a type of gene therapy which led to restored production of the Dp71 protein in the brain. They also tested the eyes of the mice and found that the signalling changes had returned to normal (Vacca *et al.* 2016). If this is also the case in people with DMD, then this type of eye testing would be a non-invasive way to tell whether a new drug therapy had restored production of dystrophin.

Dystrophin in the brain: Summary

It is likely that dystrophin is important both in the development of the brain and in its ongoing function. If future treatments can restore dystrophin in the brain in DMD, it may be possible to improve at least some of the brain-related complications in DMD. Finally, if we start to treat these complications, we will need a non-invasive way of testing that dystrophin is being produced in the brain. Using the detection of nerve signals from the retina of the eye may provide an effective way of doing this.

Conclusions

In this chapter we have discussed the ways in which the brain can be affected in DMD, and summarised the scientific research into why these differences may occur.

We have seen that several brain-related conditions can occur in DMD, including intellectual disability, ADHD, autism spectrum disorder, emotional and behavioural problems. Not everyone with DMD has these, in fact over a third of children with DMD do not experience any of these conditions. However, a third of children with DMD will have more than one of these conditions so it is important to recognise that they are at potential risk so that they can be assessed and supported from an early age.

The genetics of DMD are complex, partly because a very large gene is involved, and partly because there are many different isoforms of dystrophin, each acting in different parts of the body and in different ways. Which dystrophin isoforms are saved and which are lost in DMD depends on where the mutation is in the DMD gene. In the brain, the more dystrophin isoforms you lose, the more likely the risk of low performance in IQ tests and therefore possible learning and behaviour problems. Particularly, losing the smallest isoform of dystrophin, Dp71, can lead to more profound difficulties, although not necessarily every child with a mutation in this region of the DMD gene will have this.

The functions of dystrophin in the brain are becoming clearer, but there is still plenty that is unknown. Dystrophin almost certainly has a role both in the development of the brain and in its function throughout life, including an important role in facilitating signalling between nerve cells. However, teasing apart exactly what this means for the child with DMD is difficult at this stage.

In the future, better therapies that can target nerve cells in the brain may be able to improve some, or all, of the brain-related co-morbidities experienced by people with DMD. In the meantime, there is action that can be taken now if a child is identified with any of these difficulties. A full psychological evaluation and assessment of the child's learning and behaviour needs will identify useful interventions that can lead to improvements in the daily life of children and families affected by DMD.

Chapter Two

WHAT ARE THE LEARNING AND BEHAVIOR RISKS IN DMD?

Veronica Hinton

When living with Duchenne muscular dystrophy (DMD), there are a myriad of things to think about to try and ensure the child's best overall quality of life. Once given the diagnosis, the natural inclination is to focus on the child's medical needs to help maintain physical strength and good health. Yet, DMD may impact other areas that are just as crucial to consider for the child's (and family's) well-being. DMD is associated with increased risk of learning and behavior problems, and although not all individuals affected with DMD will have these problems, understanding what they are is imperative to ensuring each child feels comfortable with himself and enjoys his life to the fullest.

Learning and behavior concerns arise in different ways. The underlying etiology of the disorder is known to impact the brain, as well as muscle. Mutations that result in missing dystrophin from the muscle also may result in missing dystrophin isoforms from the brain. Those isoforms likely contribute to optimum brain function, and without them, children sometimes have learning and behavioral problems (to understand this in greater depth, please see Chapter 1). Behavior problems can also arise from the child and family's reaction to the disorder. Living with a neuromuscular disorder can be difficult and stressful, and people may have psychosocial difficulties that manifest as a result of struggling to adjust to the impact of the diagnosis. Additionally, educational and social opportunities may be limited as a consequence of restrictions imposed by decreased mobility. It is crucial to identify and address learning and behavior problems early, to prevent worsening over time.

Scientific research has examined learning and behavior among groups of individuals with DMD, and certain areas have been found to be susceptible to difficulty. Across studies, there is some variability in the findings, reflecting methodological differences. Yet some findings appear to be consistent. It is essential to note that although having the diagnosis of DMD may make the possibility of such problems more likely (than if the person did not have DMD), it does not mean that every child diagnosed with DMD will have the problems. Rather, the research highlights areas of possible concern.

As a parent or teacher, your individual child or student is the child who has your attention, and he is – of course – a unique individual who has distinctive characteristics. Some characteristics may be charming and delightful, others challenging, others quirky, but all part of his singular personality. Understanding whether these characteristics may be related to his DMD can help you appreciate how best to work with the issues.

This chapter will provide case studies that highlight areas of potential concern, review the findings from the studies, consider how those findings might be translated into 'real-life' situations, and whether the evidence indicates the findings are likely due to underlying etiology or reactive responses. Regardless of the cause of the problems found, all of them can be addressed and ameliorated by early identification and appropriate interventions and treatment.

■ CASE 1

Christopher, aged 7, is a very cute, sandy-haired little boy who is in the second grade. His parents have been called in by his teacher repeatedly, because she states that Christopher does not pay attention or finish his work. Christopher's teacher feels he is 'not trying'. Moreover, Christopher often gets up from his seat and walks around, disrupting other children's lessons. When he walks, his unusual posture is apparent; he has a broad-gait and arched back and he sticks his abdomen forward. Christopher's teacher notes that he has learned his alphabet, but is still unable to state the sounds that go with each letter and he cannot sound out basic words. If she tells him multi-step instructions (such as 'sit at your desk, take out your book and turn to page 5'), he may sit at his desk but then neglect to do the other things she said. Sometimes, when asked a complex question, Christopher repeats backs the last few words instead of answering.

His mother describes Christopher as 'a good kid, but maddening at times'. She reports that Christopher often does not do as she asks, and she gets frustrated with him. His father states that Christopher doesn't seem to care about his schoolwork. He knows he's bright because Christopher can tell him everything about the planets, or Star Wars, or how planes work, and he is clearly learning lots of information. Christopher's mother describes homework-time as 'horrible'. When she tries to help Christopher with his homework, Christopher often refuses to start, then rushes through and gets very upset when he is told he did something wrong, and may tantrum. In the mornings, Christopher's parents feel like they are repeatedly yelling at him to get ready for school, and every day he seems uncertain of what he is supposed to do to get out of the house, and his parents need to continually remind him. Once in bed, Christopher likes to be read to, but gets angry when his parents ask him to try and read or sound-out words.

Christopher's story reflects much of what we know about learning and behavior in DMD. On a standardized test he is found to have average intellectual function, with strengths in visual reasoning and weaker verbal skills. Most children with DMD have been shown to have IQs in the normal range, and lower verbal than nonverbal performance has been a consistent finding. As a group, children with DMD have been shown to have a distribution of IQs that are shifted down from the general population about one standard deviation, yet the majority of children with DMD do not score within the impaired range (Cotton, Voudouris, and Greenwood, 2001; Snow, Anderson, and Jakobson, 2013). This means that the majority of children with Duchenne have specific rather than global learning difficulties and should respond well to appropriate learning interventions.

As well, these findings of downward shifts of scores on tests of cognitive skills are seen even among very young children with DMD

(Connolly *et al.* 2013; Connolly *et al.* 2014; Pane *et al.* 2013). Studies that have worked with infants and toddlers with DMD giving them early developmental assessments have found that the young children score about a standard deviation lower than expected on tests of cognitive, language and motor skills. And like their older counterparts, the data are distributed such that there is a range of performance among individuals in the groups. These findings highlight that the cognitive and language delays are due to changes on the level of the brain that impact on early learning and acquisition of skills.

Christopher's difficulty answering complex questions or following multi-step instructions may well be related to underlying language difficulties. Christopher's language problems are not readily evident in his day to day life, as he converses with others clearly. During his evaluation, however, difficulties were found. On language tests, Christopher had excellent knowledge of vocabulary words and good expressive speech, but poor comprehension of complex sentences and multi-step instructions. This is best exemplified by his performance on a test that required him to accurately respond to increasing levels of verbal information. Specifically, when shown an array of different colored circles and squares, he had no difficulty accurately following the instructions to 'point to the blue circle' or 'point to the red square'. When instructions increased to the include size, he again accurately responded to instructions such as 'point to the large green circle', or 'point to the small yellow square'. As instructions increased to 'point to the red circle and the green square', Christopher began to make some errors. And when they increased to 'point to the large red square and the small blue circle', his responses looked almost random and he quickly pointed to two items. Across the early, shorter trials, he performed well, but on the later more complex trials he made multiple mistakes, and his performance was lower than what is expected for his age. Although he clearly demonstrated that he understood all the individual parts of the instructions, once they exceeded a certain length, he appeared unable to comprehend the information accurately. This illustrates that he grasps the fundamentals of language including language production, and understanding verbal concepts; however, he has a limited capacity to the amount of verbal information he can process.

Scientific research has demonstrated that, among groups of boys with DMD, language skills have been shown to be relatively weak, when compared to nonverbal skills (Billard et al. 1992; Billard et al. 1998; Bresolin *et al.* 1994; Fabbro *et al.* 2007; Hinton *et al.* 2001; Karagan, Richman and Sorensen 1980). Importantly, however, not all language skills are limited. Children have been consistently shown to have strong receptive vocabularies and good knowledge of vocabulary with limited complex receptive skills (Cyrulnik *et al.* 2008; Hinton *et al.* 2007a; Marini et al. 2007). If shown four pictures and given a word, boys with DMD can readily indicate the correct picture for a word. In contrast, if given a series of instructions, such as 'first point to this picture and then that one', their performance drops significantly. If asked to repeat a sentence back verbatim, they often neglect to say words or paraphrase what they heard. Yet, when given a word and asked to use it in a good sentence, they can generally come up with complete sentences using the word appropriately. They do not have a generalized language deficit, but instead struggle with aspects of verbal processing. Overall, boys with DMD develop many language skills well, yet there are select areas that are weak and that may not be obvious, unless specifically tested. And those areas may interfere with their daily lives in significant ways, such that they may appear not to be attending or trying, when in fact they may not be understanding all that is being said.

Additionally, studies have shown that, even among young children with DMD who are not intellectually delayed, performance on language tests tends to be depressed across most all language measures, and the profile of language performance is much less selective than that observed in older children with DMD (Chieffo *et al.* 2015; Cyrulnik *et al.* 2008; Sollee *et al.* 1985). One word receptive skills again tend to be relative strengths, but delays in both expressive speech and verbal comprehension are commonplace.

Children with DMD have also been shown, as a group, to have poor working memory (Anderson, Routh and Ionasescu 1988; Billard *et al.* 1992; Hinton *et al.* 2000; Hinton *et al.* 2001; Leaffer, Fee and Hinton 2016; Whelan 1987; Wicksell *et al.* 2004). This is most commonly tested with a digit span task; when asked to listen to and repeat back a series of digits either verbatim or in the reverse order than they were presented, children with DMD consistently do more poorly than expected for their age, when compared to their siblings, or when compared to children with other neuromuscular disorders. This difficulty with working memory is difficult to tease apart from the complex language comprehension difficulties referred to above, because in both tasks ability to attend to the verbal information, process it and then respond correctly is necessary. In real life, it again presents as the child not responding, or not responding accurately, to verbal instructions, which may give the appearance of 'not trying,' 'not caring,' or 'not listening.'

For Christopher, when asked to repeat digits forward or backwards, he says fewer than expected, and his performance looks like that of a child about two years younger. As in the test with colored shapes described above, Christopher cannot hold on to as much linguistic information as his peers. It may be that children with DMD have limited storage space for 'strings' of verbal information, such that they may not be able to 'get' lengthy statements (even though they can understand the individual parts). Not following instructions often leads to Christopher getting negative feedback from his teacher and parents, which, in turn, may lead to decreased frustration tolerance and negative self esteem with time. Providing short step-by-step verbal instructions and clear statements may be a simple intervention that can help avoid these problems.

Interestingly, during his evaluation, Christopher did well on some memory tests but struggled on others. When asked to listen to a list of words and recall as many as he could, he was at first reluctant to try and said only one word after hearing the list the first time. But with repetitions of the list, his recall improved, and his overall performance was appropriate for his age. Similarly, he had no difficulty remembering where a pattern of dots was placed on a grid, and with repeat viewings, his performance improved. For both the list learning task and the dot task, Christopher retained the information he learned over a delay, demonstrating solid memory skills. In contrast, when asked to listen to a story and then say it back, Christopher gave a few disjointed details rather than a coherent narrative, and his performance was lower than expected given his intellectual level. This likely reflected the same difficulties as seen on language tests; the verbal information in a lengthy story may have exceeded Christopher's capacity to process it all. After a delay, he recalled most of the same details that he had stated the first time, reflecting intact memory.

Research looking at memory skills among boys with DMD has been mixed, although a number of studies have demonstrated good rote learning over time with repetition (Hinton *et al.* 2001; Hinton *et al.* 2004; Wicksell *et al.* 2004). This strength offers learning strategies that children can rely on. In contrast, memory tasks studies where the children with DMD do more poorly generally reflect tasks where information is presented only once and then they are asked to recall the information. For example, Christopher only heard the stories presented one time, and he recalled fewer details than expected. This limited recall may well be related to his limited ability to attend to and process verbal information or the proposed limited verbal storage space that impacts how much verbal information can be held at any one time. Since Christopher was able to remember information he learned over a delay, his poor performance does not reflect a memory problem, but likely illustrates that he did not 'get' all the information when it was presented. Repeating statements and instructions may be a simple and effective way to help Christopher follow what he is being asked to do.

On academic testing, Christopher's reading was below grade level and his standard score on the reading tests was significantly lower than his overall IQ score. On a single word reading task, he correctly read 'in', 'cat' and 'go', but said 'car' for 'cow' and 'stop' for 'shop'. When asked to try and sound-out nonsense words, he was unable to accurately read 'mib' or 'ik,' saying instead 'my' and 'kite'. Christopher had very limited decoding skills, such that although he visually recognized some high frequency words accurately, he was unable to sound-out unfamiliar words. His errors often seem as though he is providing words that look similar to the target word, rather than trying to sound the words out. As well, Christopher did not recognize rhyming words; when asked to choose which picture from an array rhymed with 'star' he pointed to the moon rather than the car, and when asked to find the picture that rhymed with 'cat' he chose the dog, rather than the hat. This reflects limited phonological awareness. For Christopher, familiarity with his alphabet and his correct reading of some words likely relies on his strong visuo-spatial understanding, as he was very good at matching abstract shapes to each other. Interventions targeted at improving his phonological awareness such as having a parent read out loud or playing an audio book while he practices segmenting the words into phonemes will help him develop his reading skills.

Children with DMD have been shown, as a group, to have significant difficulties learning to read (Astrea *et al.* 2015; Billard *et al.* 1998;

Hendriksen and Vles 2006; Hinton *et al.* 2004). They have been found to have poor phonological abilities, (the ability to work with individual speech sounds), which contributes to difficulties learning letter-sound correspondence and decoding skills (Astrea *et al.* 2015). As such, they struggle to learn the basic mechanics of reading. And this struggle often proves to be highly frustrating, such that many children do their utmost to avoid having to read things. Some may learn to sight read high frequency words, but mastering the ability to read phonetically can be a challenge. Once they do master those skills, they may still read more slowly than their peers and have a harder time comprehending what they have read. Reading may be effortful and focused on the basic mechanics, such that it is hard for them to get the meaning from the text. Thus, children with DMD often present as having dyslexia (reading disability) and benefit from interventions that have been found to be helpful for others with dyslexia. One study examined the benefits of working with a synthetic phonics program and reported very positive results, indicating that the reading difficulties that the boys with DMD may struggle with can be ameliorated with appropriate, focused intervention that is engaging (Hoskin and Fawcett 2014) (for more information about this, please see Chapter 4).

In reviews of parent responses on questionnaires, the research has found that they report their sons with DMD often have attention problems (Banihani *et al.* 2015; Hendriksen and Vles 2008; Pane *et al.* 2012; Steele *et al.* 2008). Difficulty paying attention, not following instructions, being easily distractible and avoiding effortful tasks (all things that Christopher was noted to struggle with) are all characteristics associated with attention deficit hyperactivity disorder. Yet, some of these characteristics are also similar to the language comprehension and verbal working memory difficulties described above, and the avoidance of effortful tasks is common among children with academic difficulties in general (no one likes to take on things that they feel they may fail at!). It may be difficult to tease apart what causes what, but what is known is that children with DMD may appear inattentive and forgetful, and that can be difficult for the child, teacher and parents.

For Christopher, during the evaluation he was generally attentive to the pictures and puzzles, but became fidgety and distracted when asked questions. On those measures, he frequently asked how many more he had to do before he would be finished. In addition, when he was asked to do academic worksheets with spelling or math problems, he rushed through, sometimes writing answers without seeming to have looked at, let alone thought about, the problem. He responded very well to gentle redirection and reinforcement (e.g. when told to keep going to the end and then he would receive a sticker, he kept at the tasks). In addition, he responded very well when shown how much time was left before he received a break, and he persevered and independently checked the clock, without repeatedly asking when it would be over.

Parents have also reported more executive difficulties in children with DMD (Donders and Taneja 2009). Executive skills are those involved in oversight and planning and reflect how well a child may regulate, organize and manage his behavior and the tasks that he is supposed to do. There is overlap with the above mentioned difficulties, such that this may reflect inattention, increased distractibility and poor working memory. Other executive difficulties reported included a greater likelihood of the child with DMD having poor behavioral control (such as a 'quick fuse', or getting more upset than the situation might warrant), difficulties with transitions (trouble moving easily from one activity to another), or a rigid approach to a task (difficulty coming up with alternative strategies to solve a problem). These behaviors can be very challenging for all. Indeed, when parents with children with DMD were asked to rate their levels of stress, those with children who they rated as having high levels of behavioral problems rated themselves as dealing with significantly more stress than parents of children with few behavioral problems (Nereo, Fee and Hinton 2003). Even more striking was that the parents' stress levels were associated primarily with the child's behavior, not the child's level of physical impairment. This finding highlights the real importance of identifying and treating learning and behavioral problems for the well-being of the whole family. Participation in parent-training programs may prove to be useful for parents to help them understand and address cognitive difficulties. The use of consistent rewards such as praise and behavior charts or stickers for younger children can be helpful. However, as you will read in Chapter 5, a different way of supporting problematic behavior can be more beneficial so that young people can start to develop strategies themselves.

The scientific research has also shown areas of strength for boys with DMD. Rote learning skills and learning of factual information are areas where boys may excel (Hinton *et al.* 2001; Hinton *et al.* 2007a). Christopher's knowledge of planets, Star Wars and planes is impressive. Finding topics of interest and encouraging children to become experts in those topics may give them tremendous satisfaction, as well as ways to shine among their peers. After all, being the kid who can answer all Star Wars-related questions may prove to be a huge boost among classmates who want to know more!

■ CASE 2

Garrett, a 4-year-old preschooler with dark curls and large eyes, is described as liking to 'do his own thing'. He looks physically fit, and has large calf muscles that look like those of an athlete. Yet Garrett tires easily when walking and he prefers to play on his own in his room than play outdoors or at the park with other children. When Garret was 3 years old, his pediatrician recommended speech therapy because Garret only spoke in single words. Since then, his vocabulary has expanded dramatically. He names pictures of common items and speaks in sentences of two to three words. For example, Garrett says, 'ride on bus' and 'want more'.

Garrett likes to play with his buses, and can keep himself occupied for hours, arranging his toy buses. Garrett has special places on the shelves for his buses and he gets upset when they are rearranged or moved. His mother finds this surprising, because, in general, she notes that Garrett is careless with his clothes and other possessions, and his room 'looks like a tornado hit it'. At home, he is affectionate with his parents, and is responsive to their cuddles. Yet, when he is on his own playing, he does not seek them out to join him or show them what he has done. His parents love his huge smile and excitement when they go to the bus depot and look at the buses, and every time they get in the car, Garrett exclaims, 'Bus depot! Bus depot!' repeatedly.

At his preschool, Garrett may play next to his classmates, yet rarely with them, and he prefers to play with the buses and cars than the other items. When it is circle time, he often does not want to stop playing and join the group. Because of a few incidents where he yelled at length when the teacher tried to take away his toy and guide him to the circle, his teachers now allow him to play on his own. They note that he is not disruptive when he is on his own and seems content.

When evaluated, Garrett's overall IQ score and performance across most of the tests given was in the intellectually delayed range. He struggled on tests of both expressive and receptive language. He did correctly identify and name familiar objects (e.g. when shown a ball, pencil, watch, toy dog and toy car, he accurately identified each when he heard the word and he was able to name the object when he was shown it). Testing on more complex language tests was discontinued after multiple attempts; when asked a question about a picture, he often said 'no' and pushed away the picture books he was shown; when asked how old he was, or to repeat two-word phrases, he said nothing. In addition, Garret did not complete puzzles, identify which two items from an array went together or choose the correct picture to complete a sequence. However, Garrett did relatively well on a visual matching test showing which two items from a group went together (such as correctly choosing the circle from a group of shapes when shown a circle, and choosing the triangle when shown a triangle).

Garrett's low intellectual function and impaired language skills reflect research findings among boys with DMD. Although, as previously noted, most boys with DMD do not have intellectual delays, more boys with DMD have intellectual delays than the general population. Overall, IQ in the DMD group is distributed similarly to the general population, but it is shifted down about one standard deviation, such that a greater number of individuals' scores will fall in the intellectually delayed range (Cotton, Voudouris and Greenwood 2001; Ogasawara 1989). The research has suggested as many as one-third of children diagnosed with DMD may score two or more standard deviations below the general population on standardized tests of intelligence.

During the evaluation, Garrett had no difficulty separating from his mother. He looked at the clinician fleetingly. When she smiled at him, he did not smile back, nor did he give her a high five when she put her hand up and congratulated him. When she rolled a ball to him and encouraged him to roll it back, Garrett just held the ball. When she took out toy cars, Garrett showed interest, and smiled, but when she tried to have him drive his car on the same track where she drove hers, he instead took all the cars out of the box and parked them neatly next to the track. When she tried to put them back in the box, he became upset. At the end of the evaluation, Garrett smiled when he saw his mother and gave her a hug, but he did not say or wave good-bye to the clinician.

Garrett's poor language in combination with his limited social reciprocal skills, and rigid or stereotyped behaviors is suggestive of a diagnosis of autism spectrum disorder. Among children with DMD, autism is more commonplace than among children in the general population. Retrospective reviews of clinic populations and parent reports have indicated rates of 3 to 19 percent of children with DMD may have autism spectrum disorder (Banihani *et al.* 2015; Darke *et al.* 2006; Hinton *et al.* 2009; Wu *et al.* 2005). Standardized parent interviews of a population of 85 research participants found as many as 16 met criteria for the diagnosis (Hinton *et al.* 2009). Although some who were diagnosed were intellectually delayed, many were not. Characteristics of autism spectrum disorder in DMD can occur across intellectual levels. Garrett will benefit from standard interventions given to children with autism spectrum disorder. This might include daily behavioral guidance using applied behavior analysis techniques, speech and language therapy and social skill remediation.

Additionally, the research has shown that although most children with DMD do not have autism spectrum disorder, many have some traits that are often associated with it. For example, on parent questionnaires, parents often endorse social problems as an area of weakness for their sons (Bushby *et al.* 2001; Darke *et al.* 2006). Likewise, the above mentioned executive skill deficits that parents endorsed, such as limited mental flexibility and difficulty with transitions may be more subtle manifestations of serious problems often associated with autism spectrum disorder (Donders and Taneja, 2009). Mild difficulties with correctly understanding facial expression of different emotions has also been shown in a group of boys with DMD of normal intellectual function who were compared to their siblings (Hinton *et al.* 2007b). For some, guidance and training with executive and organizational skills may be helpful and others may benefit from participation in social skill building groups.

CASE 3

Amir, aged 11, lives with his mother, father and two brothers. He is the eldest child, short for his age and handsome. Amir attends the sixth grade. He walks slowly and cautiously, often reaching out to the wall to support himself. His school performance is average, and his teachers describe him as a quiet and studious boy. They note that recently he has seemed to be 'in a world of his own'. At school, Amir takes art classes instead of gym, but otherwise his curriculum is comparable to his peers. At lunch, he used to spend time with a group of boys and trade Pokemon cards, but now he often chooses to study on his own. Amir rarely asks for help. His manner is somewhat withdrawn, and his teachers note that when they have asked him whether he is OK, he always answers that he 'is fine', and has 'no problems'.

Amir's parents relate that he is a skilled artist. They note that he has always enjoyed building with LEGO and can build even the most complicated models. According to his parents, Amir now spends less time drawing and building with his LEGO. As well, they report he plays less with his brothers than he used to, but they think that is because they tend to play outside, and Amir is more of a 'homebody'.

Amir's parents insist that they do not discuss his physical difficulties. They do not want to worry him, or his brothers, about the seriousness of the disorder. Although they ensure that he gets good medical treatment, and have told him that his daily stretching and medication are necessary for him to 'stay well', they do not want him to get physical therapy at school because they do not want him to 'stand out'. Similarly, they share they are not yet ready to get him a wheelchair because they are worried he will feel disabled and different. They have requested their doctors not use the word 'Duchenne' for fear he will look it up on the internet and get frightened.

Amir reflects many of the strengths observed among boys with DMD; he has very strong visuo-spatial skills which allow him to draw and build very well. The scientific research has repeatedly documented that boys with DMD tend to have strengths in nonverbal, spatial skills (Cotton, Crowe and Voudouris 1998; Hinton *et al.* 2001;

Mento, Tarantino and Bisiacchi 2011; Snow, Anderson and Jakobson 2013). As well, he is bright and there are no concerns about academic difficulties, as are observed in many boys.

He is more withdrawn, interacts less with friends and his brothers, and shows diminished interest in activities he once enjoyed. Research of children with DMD has shown that depression and withdrawal are more common than in the general population, yet not seen in the majority of the children affected with DMD (Hinton *et al.* 2007b; Poysky 2007). As children get older, the risk of having depressive symptoms appears to increase. More importantly, depressive symptoms are commonly associated with poor adjustment (Elsenbruch *et al.* 2013; Poysky 2007). Across studies of children with chronic illness, depressive symptoms are more often seen among those where the parents are having difficulty coping with the disorder. Research has repeatedly shown that parents' responses to illness colors children's responses; when parents cope well with the difficulties associated with a diagnosis and are open and forthcoming about it to their children, children are more likely to adjust well (Condly 2006). The importance of speaking about DMD to your child, and how to do it, is discussed in Chapter 6.

This finding suggests that depressive symptoms are most likely a reactive response to the disorder, and not due to the underlying etiology. That means that depressive symptoms can be prevented by changes in the child's life. By treating him more as a child than patient, being open about the challenges he is facing, maximizing his social opportunities, involving him in activities he enjoys and emphasizing his strengths, parents and teachers can minimize the risk of depression in these boys. In fact, research looking at resilience among children with DMD has shown that those with better social networks and involved in more activities are less likely to have depressive symptoms (Fee and Hinton 2011).

For Amir and his family, counseling or psychotherapy would be beneficial to help him develop coping mechanisms for when he feels overwhelmed and develop ways to manage behaviors. Amir needs behavioral interventions to help lift negative moods and he likely will respond well to a cognitive behavioral therapy approach that has been shown to be effective in children with depression. This would also allow monitoring of his emotional status as self esteem can also often be an issue when faced with multiple stressors. Additionally, his parents could use help adjusting to the diagnosis and can be aided by discussing it openly in therapy. Family counseling encouraging everyone to acknowledge the illness, and all the hardships and pain it entails, and guiding them to shift their views from primarily avoidance to finding ways to feel more empowered to do what they can to change and improve things is critical. Involvement in parent organizations that encourage education and support can be helpful and rewarding. And finding ways for Amir to engage more socially and emphasizing his strengths will be useful to help improve his mood. For Amir, things like a LEGO robotics club, art classes and regular get-togethers with his friends should be encouraged.

CASE 4

Bruce, aged 16, is a heavy, good-looking teenager who is self-conscious about his 'chipmunk cheeks'. Bruce has taken Prednisone since he was 7, and his face has the typical cushingoid characteristics. Bruce used to be slim, but since he became wheelchair dependent at age 12 he has gained a significant amount of weight. He is friendly and polite and answers all questions asked of him. When asked to describe his interests, he readily discusses movies he has seen and describes his favorites articulately and animatedly. Bruce's academic performance is good. He receives As and Bs in most subjects. Bruce is conscientious about most of his studies, but says he wishes he did not have to take a foreign language because he really doesn't enjoy it.

Bruce has a group of friends who share his interests for movies and computer games. He enjoys making videos and frequently posts them online and has gotten very positive feedback. He entered one film he made into a student contest and won first place. Bruce attends a public school and is in the eleventh grade. He feels shy and awkward around girls. He plans to go to college and hopes to study law to become a civil rights lawyer.

Bruce, first and foremost, stands out as a typical teenager. He has friends and interests, socializes, studies hard, has plans for his future and is self-conscious about his looks and awkward around girls. His DMD is secondary to those characteristics. He lives with it, but continues to engage fully and enjoy his life. Not only is he a typical teenager, he reflects what the research shows can be the norm for children with DMD.

Research studies have suggested that some of the concerns that are problematic when children are younger may lessen with time (Cotton, Voudouris and Greenwood 2005; Hinton *et al.* 2016). Language problems diminish, and parents are less likely to report attention and executive skill problems among older boys (Poysky 2007). Although reading problems could potentially worsen with time without adequate interventions, children with dyslexia who receive proper interventions make notable gains in their reading abilities (Galuschka *et al.* 2014). Bruce's dislike for foreign languages may reflect some of the weaker phonological skills referred to earlier. Oftentimes, poor phonological skills not only contribute to difficulty reading but also may manifest as difficulty learning a second language (Engel de Abreu and Gathercole 2012).

Depressive symptoms have also been shown to increase with age, but as discussed above, are much less likely to occur in boys with active and engaging lifestyles (Elsenbruch *et al.* 2013; Fee and Hinton 2011; Rahbek *et al.* 2005). Bruce's love of movies and making videos and playing computer games again reflects the visuo-spatial strengths seen among boys with DMD, and these are areas that he has honed and become proficient in. Bruce's interest in civil rights is inspired in part by his own challenges navigating life in a wheelchair. And, given that study for a law degree relies on acquisition of lots of factual information, a skill that is often a strength for boys with DMD, he is in a good position to excel in his career choice.

Summary and discussion

Boys with DMD are at increased risk for learning and behavioral problems, and the areas that may be problematic have been identified through careful research. In general, language skills are more often involved than nonverbal skills, and complex receptive skills and verbal working memory may be the most susceptible to impairment. Interestingly, when skills are looked at across a group of boys with

DMD who range from intellectually impaired to superior intellectual skills, performance on tests that rely on attending to verbal information tend to be weakest, regardless of IQ (Hinton *et al.* 2000). And research evidence has shown a strong association between verbal working memory and academic achievement as well as the development of self esteem (Gathercole *et al.* 2006). For the extremely bright boy with DMD, his relative weaknesses may be inconsequential because, although weaker than his other skills, this ability is still well within the normal range, and he is better able to compensate for any weaknesses he may have. In contrast, for the child whose intellectual skills are lower, depressed abilities in attending to verbal information may have serious consequences. In addition, if boys with DMD develop verbal memory skills at a slower rate than they develop other skills it might account for why greater language difficulties are seen at younger ages.

The different areas of potential risk are likely interrelated. Difficulties with language comprehension, verbal working memory, attention, executive functions, reading and social skills may be a constellation of characteristics associated with the diagnosis of DMD. Yet, although some boys with DMD may have all of them and many challenges in their learning (such as Garrett), others may only have a few that interfere with their optimal performance (such as Christopher), and many boys will not be limited in any way by these learning risks (such as Amir and Bruce). Difficulties with emotional adjustment to living with DMD may also be observed (such as Amir) given the many potential stressors related to living with a chronic illness. What is imperative to know is that early identification and addressing any concerns that may be seen will contribute to improved lives for everyone involved.

While the list of risks is substantial, the list of strengths is as well. Nonverbal skills, such as visual reasoning, construction, and spatial understanding are areas where boys can excel. In addition, boys with DMD have been shown to have good rote memories and learn well with repetition. These skills can help augment learning and define each child's special areas of interest that may help guide him on his career path. It is important to keep in mind that every child is unique with specific strengths that should be fostered and utilized to overcome weaknesses. Although there are many stressors associated with DMD, it is important to try to focus on what is going right in a child's life and provide a supportive atmosphere at home. Studies have shown that family hardiness, caregiver health and family support all are associated with better coping and functioning within the family which benefited the child with DMD (Chen 2008; Chen and Clark 2007, 2010).

It is recommended that children with DMD receive neuro-psychological evaluations should any concerns arise, and/or at the start of school (Bushby *et al.* 2010). Every boy is unique and the standardized evaluations will allow for careful determination of whether he is having any cognitive or behavioral difficulties. Such evaluations may be useful across the age span – from preschoolers struggling with early language development to school-aged children struggling with academics to young adults struggling with job and life demands – and may be helpful to have every couple of years to document progress. Individual tailored recommendations to the problems a boy may be experiencing will ensure they do not adversely affect him.

Chapter Three

THE PHYSICAL MANAGEMENT OF DMD IN SCHOOL, COLLEGE AND BEYOND

Lianne Abbot and Victoria Selby

Introduction

As physiotherapists with considerable experience of working with children with DMD, we know that diagnosis can be a daunting and unsure time. We aim to alleviate some myths and make the journey through DMD a positive one. While we know DMD follows a general pathway, it is really important that each child and family are treated as individual, with treatments and interventions personalised to their specific needs. Different children will be affected in different ways and will need various inputs at different times. As professionals we are guided by a child's/family's needs and experiences alongside a working knowledge and good understanding of the condition. The ultimate aim is to enable anyone affected by DMD to achieve their full potential and have a happy and fulfilled life.

Aims of physiotherapy

With DMD physiotherapy the aim is to encourage a lifestyle full of activity and to minimise the impact of potential complications. This includes maintaining movement, symmetry (including scoliosis prevention), strength and fitness and slowing down the decline in function as much as possible. Other aims include pain reduction and falls management, with the overall aim of promoting best quality of life, as well as the management of respiratory complications, education and liaison.

The known pattern of DMD shows that it is a progressive condition affecting muscles, which affects movement and functions of the body with increased difficulties in carrying out activities of daily living (Fujiwara *et al.* 2009). Medical interventions such as steroids and regular monitoring of the heart have changed the natural history of DMD resulting in longer life expectancy and boys achieving much more. Intensive global research and many clinical trials are being carried out focusing on either further understanding the natural history of DMD (natural history studies) or improving the outcome of DMD. Alongside the research there is an increasing need for physiotherapy input. In order for boys with DMD to reach their maximum potential and fully participate in life it is essential that their physical abilities are optimised.

Current challenges

One of the greatest challenges with physiotherapy and for everyone involved is the communication between specialist centres, local centres, schools and families. There are many reasons for this. Therapy provision for DMD in the UK is part of the National Standards of Care; however, there are huge variations in provision throughout the country and ultimately the world, meaning children with DMD in different areas get varied physiotherapy provision. With regular shifts in government policy and NHS changes, the demand on time and money is increasing and can mean reduced input. However, we hope that this chapter will help you understand the importance of physiotherapy and how as parents and teachers you can support it to happen.

Impact of steroids

Currently steroid treatment is the best and most common treatment for DMD and is keeping boys walking and more active for longer, on average for about three more years (Henricson *et al.* 2013). Steroids increase strength, decrease falls and improve breathing function. This can have a positive impact on well-being and bone and spine health and may prolong walking long enough to reduce likelihood or severity of scoliosis (Henricson *et al.* 2013).

However this treatment regime does not come without its side effects. The main side effects for the consideration of the physiotherapist are increased appetite, leading to weight gain, and the effects on bone density. The use of steroids can be a difficult decision; however, the benefits often outweigh the negatives.

If a child with an underlying muscle weakness condition, such as DMD, has a rapid increase in weight gain or a higher than average weight, they will find it even more difficult to move. This is essentially because they have more body to move. Due to the use of steroids, boys are often delayed in reaching puberty and their height can be affected. They tend to have shorter limbs and trunk with increased mass, which makes movement more biomechanically challenging.

Reduced weight bearing exercise and long term use of steroids have a known side effect of reducing bone density (Quinlivan *et al.* 2005). Referral to an endocronologist can lead to regular monitoring and medication that can help counter bone density issues. In addition, there are weight bearing exercises and activities that can not only help physical functioning but also have a positive impact on maintaining good bone health, (Jansen *et al.* 2010).

What to expect in a physiotherapy assessment

Boys in the UK will be routinely seen at a specialist centre every six months for an outpatient clinic appointment. They will have local input to monitor and support activities at school and home.

Assessment at a specialist centre includes:

- joint range of movement – contractures, asymmetry, hyper-mobility

- muscle power

- North Star Assessment: a functional outcome measure looking at the boys' abilities to do tasks such as rising from the floor, standing on one leg, hopping, jumping and completing a step and how they do this (i.e. any compensations)

- 10 metre timed test and gait/walking assessment

- timed rise from the floor

- six-minute walk test

- spine and neck assessment

- assessment of the need for orthosis and equipment such as wheelchairs, etc.

If boys are on research trials then other outcome measures may be used as well.

These assessments are conducted to allow comparison and accurate assessment of changes which then impact on recommendations and treatment. Not all aspects need to be completed at each assessment if there are any difficulties; it is just a snapshot to see how the child is doing. Talking to the family to determine what is going on at home can be just as helpful, so do not worry if your child doesn't show all of their abilities on the day.

Other tests which may be completed during the specialist centre assessment include: sleep study, heart monitor – ECHO, lung function and respiratory assessment.

DMD in the different age groups

We will now look at physiotherapy issues regarding different age groups. Of course every child with DMD is unique, but most follow a similar pattern.

4 to 7 years

It is often at school when boys' difficulties compared to their peers are first noticed and school staff may be the first to highlight these. Early difficulties include rising from the floor, running, sitting from low seats and falls.

Physiotherapy

Physiotherapy is a vital and daily essential in the boys' lives that can be done at home or school. If the child has extra support in school then their physiotherapist should be able to train their teaching assistant (TA) to complete their physiotherapy to help support the family.

Activity

Activity can be a cause for concern for parents and teachers as they fear it may cause muscle damage and speed up deterioration; in fact, the opposite is true, as exercise is of vital importance. Keeping boys active and strong is crucial to gain skills and delay the loss of ambulation and should be fun! While boys with DMD may fall more than others, it is no reason to stop them participating in fun games with their friends. Try to find ways to ensure that they can stay active and included without taking unnecessary risks that can lead to serious injury.

Activities such as swimming, cycling and walking are excellent for promoting symmetrical muscle strength, fitness and in turn the development of function/gross motor skills. For younger boys, soft play and walking over different surfaces including grass, slopes and pebbles is good for developing balance and further progressing skills as well. For older boys, activities such as kick-boxing and horse riding can be good options, and they should also be encouraged to participate fully in PE. This is a lifelong condition and promoting normal activity is much better advice than specific physiotherapy exercises. This should therefore aim to be normal and fun and can be done by all the family!

There is unproven research into weight training exercises but weights are not encouraged. Activities to avoid include rugby, trampolining (as this can cause injury and increase the risk of ankle tightness), and scooters (as these promote asymmetrical muscle use). Bikes (including balance bikes) are a much better option as they encourage symmetrical activity and promote general fitness.

The child is the best measure of how much activity they can do – do not limit this. The best physiotherapy is to encourage your child to be a normal, healthy, active child rather than wrap him in bubble wrap. Just as people who are unaffected by DMD become weaker if they do not exercise, a lack of activity will affect a child with DMD. A team in the Netherlands have explored the impact of exercise and concluded that if boys with DMD stop exercising then their physical abilities reduce, in other words they must 'use it or lose it' (Jansen *et al.* 2010). However, it is important to make sure that your child is not overdoing it; if you are concerned about this look out for haematuria (cola coloured urine) as this is a sign of muscle damage.

Inclusion in PE and games

If you are a teacher there are many helpful things you can do to include children with DMD in PE lessons. You may need to adapt some of your activities so that they will have an impact on their development. Focus on inclusion and how activities can support physical development for the whole class and in particular the child with DMD; for example, 'Penguin' or heel walking can support the stretching of ankles. The whole class can benefit from exercises that will help children with DMD – so they do not always have to be doing separate activities. Children with DMD should be active rather than just sitting during this time; often, at this age, they are able to do many of the things their peers can do. It is every child's right to participate and access PE and this can be one of their favourite parts of school. Boys should wear trainers rather than plimsoles when participating in PE, as plimsoles are not supportive.

Ankle stretches

Ankles are the most common and often the first joint to become tight, which has great functional implications. This is why physiotherapists always go on about them! Ankle tightness can lead to functional difficulties separate to muscle weakness, for example rising from the floor, chair or when completing stairs. It is therefore is vital to maintain range of movement. If you try to do these activities without letting your ankle bend you will realise how difficult it is! Once the ankle becomes tight it is very difficult to stretch as muscle becomes replaced by fat and connective tissue, accounting for calf hypertrophy (larger calf size), so prevention is better.

Ankle stretches therefore often need to be completed daily. These can be incorporated into PE and games, with the other children in the class completing them too to help reduce exclusion, or they can be completed at home. Routine is often best and an effective way of fitting them into normal life, for example, when brushing their teeth as this means two minutes of stretching built in. TAs can be trained by the local physiotherapist to follow a programme that is recommended for the specific child.

Active stretches (which the child does himself) are generally best. Examples include the classic footballers' stretch (see Figure 3.1) or standing on a pile of books (see Figure 3.2). In this stretch make sure the heels are on the floor, keeping the toes facing forwards. The books should be high enough to feel a stretch at the back of the ankle. This can be done as a game or while watching TV or playing computer games. If the child feels wobbly, they can stand next to something stable to hold onto.

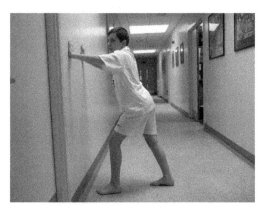

Figure 3.1 Active ankle stretch.

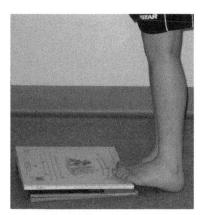

Figure 3.2 Active ankle stretch.

Depending on the age and understanding of the child, stretches may need to be active assisted (with you helping them a bit). Passive stretches (just done by the parent or teacher) can be difficult, as the child will often fight against them. In the stretch shown in Figure 3.3, encouraging the child to pull their toes ('toes towards their nose') up to help with this is more effective as well as working the dorsiflexor (pulling up) muscles which do not get much activity, making this active assisted.

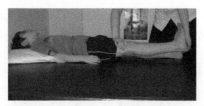

Figure 3.3 Active assisted ankle stretch.

Place one hand on the sole of their foot, cupping the heel. Try to keep the child's toes facing upwards as much as possible. Hold the knee straight with the other hand but do not push it down. Gently, but firmly, increase the stretch that the child has started. Mild to moderate resistance should be felt but you should never push through strong resistance. No pain should be felt.

Other joints may get tight, for example, long finger flexors and supination (turning the hand over), and may need stretching as well, your physiotherapist can advise. This can be done through games that get the hand down flat, for example, playing Twister or using playdough.

Hamstring stretches

Hamstrings (the muscle down the back of your thigh) should not be actively stretched. Hamstring tightness doesn't have a big effect on function, unlike ankle tightness, and can in fact be beneficial. Hamstrings attach into the pelvis, and therefore if they are tighter they can add stability to compensate for hip extensor weakness keeping the child upright. There is also research into unaffected children and hamstring length which found a hamstring angle of 0 to 50° to be normal within different age ranges (Katz, Rosenthal and Yosipovitch 1992). It is unusual for anyone to be able to touch the floor with their legs straight – unless they are a gymnast or very flexible!

Splints

Boys with DMD often have to wear ankle foot orthosis (AFOs) to help maintain their ankle range of movement once they start to develop tightness (see Figures 3.4a and 3.4b). These should be custom-made for each child and be non-lined to minimise sweating, with breathable holes. They should have a cushioned Velcro strap, smooth edges and be set at 90°. It has been proven that AFOs alongside stretches are better than either alone (Skalsky and McDonald 2012).

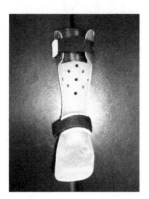 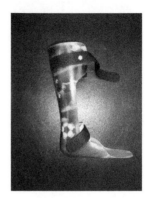

Figures 3.4a and b Night splint.

The best way to use AFOs for maintaining ankle range of movement is to wear them at night for a prolonged stretch (Skalsky and McDonald 2012). However, boys can find them uncomfortable or annoying. Wearing AFOs on alternate legs can be another option (i.e. wear one on the left one night and on the right the following), but if discomfort continues to be an issue then they may be worn for a period of time during the day, for example when watching TV or during a lesson.

AFOs should not be worn when walking. Boys with DMD walk on their toes for a reason, as explained in the next section, and wearing AFOs stops this.

AFOs should be custom made for each boy and not off the shelf. Socks can be used to minimise sweating if this is an issue, but they are non-lined and have holes, so the design should minimise this. AFOs may cause some red marks due to pressure, however, these should resolve within 30 minutes of removal. If the red marks do last longer then the AFOs should be reviewed.

Posture and Achilles Tendon (TA) tightness explanation

You may have noticed boys with DMD walking on their toes and having an increased lordosis (arched back). These changes are to compensate for patterns of weakness. The boys often toe walk and have an arched back, holding their arms back in order to bring their centre of gravity behind; their increased hamstring tightness serves to stabilise the pelvis and to enable them to keep walking.

These boys are on their toes for a reason – they may not even have tight ankles; however, this can lead to tightness which, as already mentioned, causes further functional difficulties. Walking on their toes can help boys with DMD to walk for longer and should not be discouraged when they are older. The arched back posture is not possible to address, as, again, this helps the boys walk for longer.

Wheelchair

The introduction of a manual wheelchair can be a very upsetting time for families, especially when they do not feel their son needs this. However, for the boys themselves this can often be a liberating time when they gain independence and rely less on adults to support them, giving them more freedom. Other children can often be jealous and want to have a go too! Manual wheelchairs can be difficult and timely to source, therefore it is vital that this is done early. They should be lightweight and manual so that the boys can self propel, giving them independence and an opportunity to work on their upper limb and truck strength. There are many wheelchair sports which can be played and are fun and enjoyable. Research reported by Archer and colleagues suggests that boys who self propel their wheelchair maintain a good spinal posture and therefore their lung function remains better for longer (Archer *et al.* 2016). These wheelchairs do not need to be used all the time but can be useful, for example on school trips when a lot of walking is involved, to ensure that the child is able to fully participate and access their environment.

Buggies, while looking more 'normal', are not appropriate for boys once they reach school age and should not be used as a substitute for a wheelchair as they give no independence and often promote poor posture.

Pacing

Preserving energy is important and getting the balance right means the child can have the energy to do the activities they want to. For example, if a child wants to go to the park or a birthday party it can be better to let him travel there using his wheelchair and then run around the park, instead of using up all his energy in getting there. The child can go to school in their wheelchair, but there needs to be somewhere safe to park it so that they can be supported to be active once at school.

7 to 11 years (Junior school)

Every child with DMD is different; however, it is often around this age that walking starts to become more difficult and they may lose ambulation. Boys will often present with a reduced range of movement at their ankles, more frequent falls, walking on toes and they are slower getting up off the floor.

Activity

If the child is struggling to pedal a bike, and this is something they enjoy, there are other options such as low geared or lightweight bikes. These can be purchased through charity funding as they can often be very expensive. Local physiotherapists can often arrange this or offer a trial to see if this is beneficial.

As boys with DMD start to find walking and other tasks more difficult it is really important to try to participate in activities and exercise to maintain strength and general fitness. Swimming is particularly beneficial as the buoyancy of the water allows movements that they cannot do on land, such as walking. When 'swimming' is recommended it doesn't necessarily mean doing lengths up and down a pool. Any movement in water will help, including walking forward, backward, side stepping. Also include arm movements, the water will provide some form of resistance. Regular hydrotherapy in individuals with DMD helps to maintain strength and function (Honório, Batista and Martins 2013). Swimming is an activity that the whole family can enjoy, so has the added benefit of being inclusive.

Sometimes the temperature in council run pools can be cold and access to hydrotherapy can be limited. Hotels, spas and hospices sometimes have warmer pools that can be used. The Muscular Dystrophy Support Hub lists local pools and other nearby activities.[1]

As boys with DMD start to find things more difficult, they may become more socially isolated and excluded from activities. There are many sports that are available to wheelchair users, ranging from wheelchair football to boccia. It is important to find an activity that each individual is happy to do as a hobby; ideally it should should aim to target their strengths as well as include them in leisure pursuits. Being able to participate in recreational activities, on equal terms, and

---

1   www.musculardystrophyuk.org/support-hub/services-near-you

socialise outside the home environment on a regular basis has shown to have a positive effect on perceived disease-specific, health-related quality of life (Otto *et al.* 2017).

Physiotherapy advice/treatment

When the boys start to lose ambulation, the main objective of the physiotherapist is to help maintain strength, function and independence. There is continued focus on upper limb function and the maintenance of joint range of movement (particularly of the legs). This is achieved by exercises, activities, stretching and the introduction of equipment.

Loss of ambulation

A boy with DMD will inevitably lose ambulation. Injuries, fear of falls, increased falls, weakness, increased difficulty and being different are all factors that influence walking, and ultimately loss of the ability to do this (Emery and Muntoni 2003). Often a child will fall and hurt themselves which can lead to non-ambulation (Larson and Henderson 2000).

At this stage, there are two options: Knee Ankle Foot Orthosis (KAFOs) (see Figure 3.5), or full time wheelchair use. These options need explaining and discussing with the child and their family. The transition from walking to using a wheelchair is often a relatively short time frame and a boy will generally know what is best for him. It is often a big hurdle for the family, but whichever option is taken will often be liberating for the boy. Whether it is KAFOs or a wheelchair, the child will have increased control and independence, and very often feel in charge of the decision. There is no right or wrong choice but each option needs provision of equipment.

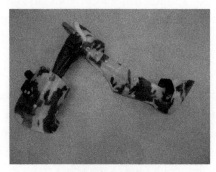

Figure 3.5 KAFO.

KAFOs

KAFO walking has a different walking pattern than that of unaided walking. KAFOs ensure that the leg is straight and the knee is unable to bend, therefore the walking pattern has more emphasis on lateral weight shift and hip hitching, rather than the usual hip and knee flexion pattern. Local physiotherapists will often trial the walking in long leg splints and monitor the child at home and in school. Gaiters are a temporary, cheaper fabric version of KAFOs which can be trialled to see if these are of benefit as they also stop the knee from bending. It is important that the gaiters are used in school and that staff are supportive and compliant with the exercise programme and advice. They should also have knowledge of the altered walking pattern to enble them to best support the child. It is hugely advocated that each child has specialist and individual support to achieve this, as this will allow optimal use and success of KAFOs. When providing KAFOs, there also needs to be a consideration for when their use should be stopped. This is often where the physiotherapist relies on information from the school and home setting. The decision to stop using KAFOs can be made for a number of reasons, including the young person or family's choice and safety.

Teachers can play an important and necessary part in the use of KAFOs. It is important for KAFOS to be worn daily and this requires the support of the school. Prior to putting them on time needs to be taken to carry out stretches. KAFOs need to be worn for a period of time in order to provide a stretch to the legs as well as to enable mobility, independence and an upright posture. Often a posterior walker (a walker that goes behind the user such as a Kaye walker, rather than the traditional Zimmer frame which goes in front) will also be used, requiring more space.

KAFOs are not suitable for every child or family, and the final decision should be taken by the family in conjunction with the medical teams.

WHEELCHAIRS

If a family decides that KAFOs are not for them, a wheelchair will be used for the majority of the time. This could either be a manual or electric one. Whichever type of wheelchair it is, it is important that the boys spend some time out of their wheelchair, as we all know sitting in the same position for a long time causes aches and pains, stiffness, as well as contractures and weakness. A wheelchair that a boy can self-propel or drive lets him have more independence. He may possibly start to explore all the places he previously struggled to get to, be warned!

Every child that is provided with an electric wheelchair should have a manual wheelchair to use as a back-up, in case of malfunction of the electric one.

As each child is different and progression varies within the DMD population, it is difficult to predict when a child will become more dependent on an electric wheelchair. They will still need changes in position, for pressure relief, but this often coincides with an increasing workload at school and increasing demands on the child's time. Electric wheelchairs provided should have the capability of tilt in space and ideally a high/low function. Tilt in space is a function that allows the child to rest back and have the beneficial effects of pressure relief.

Privately or charity funded electric wheelchairs often have many more features which can be used to achieve a change in position.

Safety can be a concern with electric wheelchairs; however, there are attendant controlled wheelchairs that can enable family members to push their child in a wheelchair as they get bigger and heavier. E-motion wheels can help boys to self-propel their wheelchair if they struggle with the strength to do this.

Introduce equipment/home adaptations to promote independence

Boys will find activities of daily living and mobility increasingly difficult as they get older (or even during a growth spurt), particularly tasks such as rising from the floor, walking/running and going up and down the stairs. In order to facilitate independence, allow the child to access their entire environment (at home and school) and for manual handling and safety reasons, equipment will be recommended.

If a child has frequent falls a Mangar riser or portable hoist will be recommended to avoid lifting the child and help prevent injury of the child and carer. Backcare, a UK charity, found that around 70 per cent of unpaid carers suffer from back pain – so be careful and adhere to manual handling advice.[2] If a hoist is provided, it should be one that lowers to the floor and the correct slings and training provided.

2   www.backcare.org.uk/i-have-back-or-neck-pain/carers

If a child is often falling at school, he will probably think it's time to start using a wheelchair more, for self-preservation. Access ramps and paths will need to be cleared and ready to use. While some wheelchairs are 'all terrain' wheelchairs, the majority are not. So pot holes need filling, steps need a ramp option and access to all areas is a must to ensure inclusion and equality.

EQUIPMENT AT SCHOOL

In addition to a hoist, other equipment will be recommended for use in school.

Wheelchairs are recommended at school to promote independence and ensure safety, as mentioned previously. In order to effectively carry out the child's physiotherapy programme, equipment such as a wide plinth or mat should be used. Often exercises can be done using items such as a standing frame, a gym ball or posterior walker. This will be guided by the local physiotherapist. Many boys report these exercises can be dull and boring, so if you are a teacher or a parent, talk to your physiotherapist about how you can make them more fun so that boys want to take part. Do them with a friend, have rewards, whatever it takes...

An occupational therapist is likely to recommend equipment that is needed in the classroom or at school and this may include a sloping board, specialist writing and/or eating utensils. The introduction of touch typing and use of a keyboard in the early stages of school life is recommended, as children may find keeping up with writing increasingly difficult. They may need help from their TA or a scribe to help them reach their full potential. This needs preplanning, particularly for exams.

EQUIPMENT AT HOME

At home it is likely that a moving bed which helps them change position themselves will be required to get a good night's sleep – which helps parents too. As a child grows older, home equipment may also include a BiPAP machine for respiratory care and a feeding pump to help with nutritional input.

THROUGH FLOOR LIFT

At school, boys with DMD will often find going up and down the stairs difficult, especially if there are other people also using the stairs and there is limited time. It is highly recommended that they are given plenty of time to move between classrooms during the school day and that they take a friend to help carry bags, etc.

Where possible, boys with DMD should have a special pass and be allowed to use a lift if there is one; under the Equality Act, 2010, they should not be excluded from specialist lessons and activities due to access or time reasons.[3]

A through floor lift at home is also necessary. Remember it is always better to start building projects early. Local authorities are currently experiencing funding crises that can slow the process down.

Other home and school adaptations that need to be considered are: ramps for wheelchair access, a wheelchair accessible toilet with grab rails and enough space.

WEE BOTTLES

Once a boy with DMD is no longer able to safely or effectively transfer from his wheelchair to the toilet, other provisions need to be made. This could include the use of a hoist and/or the provision of a urine bottle that the child can use while seated. As toileting issues can become an embarrassing subject, especially as a child gets older, it is important for the teaching staff and helpers to find a suitable solution that minimises embarrassment. Having a designated bag on the back of the wheelchair that holds a bottle, or having bottles stored for use in a disabled toilet is helpful.

If you are out and about in the UK, the Changing Places Consortium launched its campaign in 2006 on behalf of the over a quarter of a million people who cannot use standard accessible toilets. This gives users a safe and comfortable toilet, which has more space and the right equipment, including a height adjustable changing bench and a hoist.[4]

---

3   www.gov.uk/rights-disabled-person/education-rights
4   www.changing-places.org

ORTHOTICS

Specialist orthotics such as KAFOs and spinal jackets tend to be provided by specialist services. Less specialist orthotics such as night resting splints should be provided locally and monitored regularly.

Serial casting

If ankles become tight despite stretches and splints, serial casting (see Figure 3.6) can be an alternative option to surgery for improving ankle range of movement if the child's ankles cannot get to plantargrade (0 degrees or feet flat on the floor). This will not stop him walking on his toes, but can make activities such as standing still, going up or down stairs or rising from the floor or a chair easier; it can also improve tolerance to splints if they are not fitting well. Serial casting involves three plaster cast changes over two weeks, changing the casts twice a week to stretch the Achilles Tendons (often referred to as TAs). During this time the child should be encouraged to walk in their casts, if able, as this helps to stretch the ankle. They should not be on for more than two weeks, as longer than this can lead to muscle wasting. Serial casting is often successful but does depend how long the TAs have been tight for, and their level of tightness. Once this is completed it is important to continue with stretches and splints to maintain the range gained.

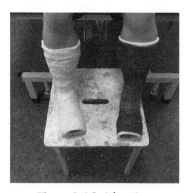

Figure 3.6 Serial casting.

Education health care plan (EHC) – help needed in PE and beyond

All children should be included in PE at school; it is not good enough to recommend wheelchair users go to the library for extra study. PE and games should be adapted to the level of each pupil and a boy with DMD should have someone to help him during these lessons.

The natural history of DMD tells us that, even when having to use a wheelchair for safer and quicker mobility, the boys continue to have good use of their arms for a much longer time period (Pane *et al.* 2014). Therefore games such as table tennis, basketball and boccia are all excellent sports that could be done. There is a plethora of sports for disabilities, and each child should have the access to practise and learn about sports within their domain.

11 to 16 years (Secondary school)

By this point the majority of boys are non-ambulant; however, it is vital that they still have an opportunity to change position and not sit in their wheelchairs all day. Other considerations when transitioning to a new school need to include access for electric wheelchairs to the school buildings, toilets, changing facilities, physiotherapy, space and 1:1 support for their individual learning and physical needs.

Stretches

Once the boys are no longer walking, stretches are of vital importance as they spend more time in a seated position. This means they are more likely to become tight in their joints. For example, if you do not stand up your hips, knees and ankles become stiffer. Boys should therefore continue with a passive stretching programme under the supervision of their physiotherapist and with help from a teaching assistant and parents. If it is no longer possible for the boys to participate in active stretching, the exercises must be completed passively. Other joints such as elbows and necks must not be forgotten as these can become stiff too. As well as stretches, splints, standing frames and activities such as swimming can help maintain range of movement.

Splints

When they are no longer ambulant, young men with DMD can choose if they would rather wear their AFOs during the day or night time. Boys can wear these under their trousers if they prefer them not to be visible. Splints still need to be worn for a prolonged period as they are needed to maintain range of movement and prevent foot deformity. Poorly positioned feet can lead to pain, pressure sores, blisters and difficulty with positioning/seating in a wheelchair.

Standing frames

Once KAFOs are no longer an option a standing frame can be beneficial if the child's muscles are not too tight to use this. A standing frame helps to maintain range of movement as joints are stretched and they are in an extended position. It also encourages weight bearing, and can aid digestion and reduce constipation. Additionally, it can have a positive impact on quality of life, as boys are able to interact with their peers at eye level.

Equipment

It is hoped by this point that the family and school will have all the relevant adaptations and equipment to reduce the manual handling risks of lifting the boys. Some of this has already been discussed in the previous section; however, there are other pieces of equipment that can encourage independence; for example, a closomat toilet. This sprays water and has an inbuilt drier, which allows boys to clean themselves after using the toilet rather than depending on someone else to clean them.

Wheelchairs and seating

By this point all boys should have an electric wheelchair if this is a safe option. They may need more support to ensure they are sitting straight, for example, a moulded seat or thoracic supports, to encourage symmetrical and supportive seating which also includes the head rest and position of the foot plates.

Scoliosis

Historically, scoliosis was a very common presentation in boys with DMD once they lost ambulation. Due to steroids, which enable better postural management and prolonged walking, the development of scoliosis is often now less severe. However, backs will still be routinely checked and monitored in clinics. When they are no longer walking, boys' risk of developing scoliosis increases as they spend more time in their chair and often lean to one side (Archer *et al.* 2016). Reducing scoliosis is important, so a good central seated position (i.e. not leaning to one side) is essential. Care should be taken when thinking about a child's seating; he may need supports on their wheelchair or a moulded backrest to help support him.

A spinal brace (also known as TLSO – Thoracic Lumbar Sacral Orthotic/jacket – see Figure 3.7) may be indicated to help prevent the deterioration of spinal posture. This should be used throughout the day when sitting but should be put on lying down with their hips and knees bent. It is not required when sleeping as gravity combined with abdominal weakness is the main cause of scoliosis.

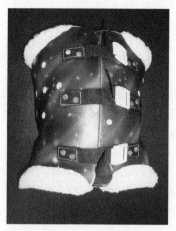

Figure 3.7 TLSO.

As well as symmetrical activities, self-propelling a wheelchair can further help to reduce the scoliosis risk. It is important that any asymmetry of ankle contractures are addressed when still ambulant as this can otherwise lead to early scoliosis.

Surgery

Sometimes surgical intervention is required to improve posture or function. Any proposed surgery requires a thorough pre-assessment and a multidisciplinary approach to ensure the least amount of stress is caused to the child and family.

Spinal surgery may be needed for scoliosis or Achilles Tendon (TA) release if the child has tight TAs. Hamstrings should never be released as this is not beneficial or effective.

Respiratory

As boys with DMD get older they are at risk of chest complications due to weak muscles (diaphragm/abdominals) and a weak cough.

This can lead to recurrent chest infections and can make secretion clearance difficult.

There are ways to pick these problems up, for example, monitoring for hypoventilation which involves looking for early morning headaches, nocturnal awakening, fear of going to sleep, difficulty waking, fatigue and difficulty concentrating.

Chest physiotherapy varies and may involve manual techniques such as percussion (to help move the secretions), assisted coughs (to help improve the cough strength), use of a LVR bag (Lung Volume Recruitment bag to give bigger breaths) or a cough assist (a machine to help give bigger breaths and cough). In many centres there are an increasing number of specialist respiratory physiotherapists to help with the management of chest complications and make respiratory difficulties less scary.

Assessment and effective management can prolong life expectancy, increase quality of life and reduce hospital admissions, which is of benefit to the young person and family – no one likes to spend more time in hospital than they need to.

And beyond

Boys with DMD are now living into adulthood and should have access to a physiotherapist in adult services, who will support them with respiratory, physical and any other issues. Some of these matters will be discussed by adults who are living with DMD in Chapter 9.

Summary

- Encourage normal activity and a normal childhood, scrapes and bruises are part of being a child.

- Physiotherapy should not over-burden the child and family with exercise programmes and stretches. It is intended to reduce the burden of care, not increase it.

- Focus stretches on areas where tightness can lead to a loss of function, cause asymmetry and affect ambulation. Don't overstretch hamstrings.

- No day splints when still ambulant.

- Plan early for equipment which will be needed both at home and school.

- Being aware of other complications and respiratory management is important.

- Physiotherapy is important but only a small part of the child's life.

Chapter Four

EARLY INTERVENTION FOR READING AND LEARNING

Janet Hoskin

Introduction

In this chapter I will share information on what we know about barriers to learning and behaviour in younger children with DMD, and what we can learn from other neuro-developmental impairments such as dyslexia. I will discuss the powerful impact we can have as parents and teachers despite the genetic basis of DMD, and I will suggest strategies and interventions that can help support children to become confident readers and learners. I will explore how children are assessed, and I will discuss the role that teaching assistants (TAs) can play to help children with DMD develop their skills and independence.

First things

It is essential to start off with the premise that our children who have DMD are going to live into adulthood. By this I am not intending to trivialise the challenges that DMD throws at us, nor am I suggesting that it isn't a life-threatening impairment that needs serious monitoring, care and support. I do mean, however, that we should be talking to our children and young people from the earliest age, as we would with any other child, about what they want to do when they grow up. We should be encouraging them to have aspirations about their future. Most children will not become professional footballers whether they have DMD or not, so we must not be afraid to help them dare to dream about the future. Becoming an adult brings with it both opportunities and responsibilities which means that our children will need to develop skills to make choices and have control in their lives. Simply allowing them to avoid schoolwork because it makes them unhappy will not prepare them for the challenges and chances ahead.

What we know about preschool children with DMD

Sometimes, learning and language difficulties stand out and are diagnosed before DMD itself (Bushby *et al.* 2010; Kaplan, Osborne and Elias 1986). Children with DMD under the age of 6 often have significantly more generalised developmental delay than other children of the same age, particularly in the areas of motor and speech skills. However, these difficulties usually become more specific as they get older so they may find particular tasks, such as reading or spelling, more challenging than other activities (Cyrulnik *et al.* 2007; Smith *et al.* 1989). It is not unusual for children with impaired motor skills to have associated cognitive impairments, for example, this has been shown to be the case in children with specific language impairment and dyslexia, and those with early speech delay can be at risk of later literacy difficulties (Bishop and Adams 1990; Nicolson, Fawcett and Dean 2001). However, this does not mean that all children with early delays in these areas will go on to have reading or learning difficulties, and what we as parents and teachers do in the early years can make a difference to their cognitive development.

Starting school

As parents of children with life-limiting impairments we may have mixed feelings about them starting school. It's a landmark point in their lives and something to be celebrated, but there are many anxieties to cope with, particularly over physical safety and friendships. The truth is that all parents are nervous about their children starting school, and at the age of 4 or 5 years children often play in parallel rather than collaboratively (Smidt 2011). Many will need support with getting dressed after PE or opening their lunch boxes, so our children will probably not appear that conspicuous compared to the rest of the class.

Nevertheless, it is essential at this time that teachers and all school staff are fully aware of the learning and behaviour risks that are associated with DMD.

Although we are not looking for extra labels for a child with DMD, we know that labels can bring support and resources that can be difficult and expensive to gain otherwise. It is what Martha Minow termed 'The Dilemma of Difference' (Minow 1985). So if your child is diagnosed as being on the autism spectrum, for example, you may gain access to extra resources and training that may support parents and teachers to gain a greater understanding of his needs; if a child has difficulties learning to read it can be useful to work with a dyslexia specialist who may be able to assess him for reading and recommend a range of interventions. From visiting lots of schools across the UK it is often evident to me that many teachers feel that they need 'permission' to intervene with a child with DMD, and are sometimes fearful of the diagnosis because it involves such serious health implications. This can sometimes mean they are reticent to refer to outside agencies or put in place something they would expect to see for any other child who was beginning to struggle in their learning.

As parents of children with DMD we are asking a lot – we want you to see our children as you would any other child who is experiencing difficulties learning to read or behave at that age, and offer appropriate assessment and intervention with the highest expectations. However, it is true that we often need you to cut him (and us) some slack if he is really struggling on a particular day. This is because children with DMD are often very tired. In the same way that a child with reading difficulties or ADHD may have bad days and be very tired simply from the sheer act of concentrating so hard in comparison with his peers for six hours, so may the child with DMD.

Genes vs. the environment

As you have learned by now, DMD is not only a neuromuscular impairment, but a neuro-developmental one. However, even though there is a genetic basis for these differences, as outlined in Chapter 1, it is important not to be genetically deterministic. Although quite old, Frith and Morten's 'Causal Modelling Framework' underlines the importance of the environment when looking at a neuro-developmental impairment (Frith 1999). This model, that is used to explain the causes of dyslexia, demonstrates a clear three-stage causal chain from biology to behaviour, showing how differences in our biological make up (genes and neurology) can cause changes in our cognitive processes (how we think and process information) that in turn impact on our behaviour (for example, how we read or communicate). However, Frith argues that the environment plays a crucial role in each of these three stages (Frith 1999).

By environment she is referring to issues regarding background, culture and education. In other words, what we do as parents and teachers to help our children develop skills can actually change the way their brains work. This is called neuro-plasticity. Nobody is born with the ability to read, and there is no identified single gene for reading: we have all had to transform the way we think and process information in order to become successful readers (The Royal Society 2011). Neuro-plasticity is illustrated in the case of London cab drivers who have to learn the 'Knowledge' (all the routes around London). It has been shown that those drivers who pass the test increase the part of their brain responsible for holding information about places and names (called the hippocampus). However, when they retire the hippocampus reduces back in size, indicating the importance of 'use it or lose it' (Woolett, Spiers and Maguire 2009). Not only does this suggest the effect education and learning can have on the brain, it also points to the importance of focused practice in order to develop expertise in any skill (Ericsson and Pool 2017)

We know that the brain is more 'plastic' (changeable) when we are younger, and so it is easier to learn new skills at that time, especially those such as learning a new language (The Royal Society 2011). Therefore, early intervention in reading and learning is always advised. Additionally, as we grow older we often become more aware of failure if something is challenging, and so we have to overcome our self-doubt and lack of confidence (Alexander-Passe 2006; Stanovich 1986).

What causes children to experience reading difficulties?

The most documented causal theory of reading difficulties over the past 40 years is phonological deficit (Snowling 2000; Stanovich 1996).

This means a difficulty in distinguishing and manipulating sounds and consequently in blending them together to make words, for example, putting 'c' with 'a' and 't' to make 'cat'. Children with phonological difficulties may also struggle to hear rhymes, remember song lyrics or break up words that they hear into chunks or sounds for example 'football' into 'foot' and 'ball' (Bradley and Bryant 1983; Vellutino *et al.* 2004).

Other researchers have suggested that as well as being able to distinguish different sounds, many young people with dyslexia-type difficulties struggle with processing the sounds and language that they hear (Wolf and Bowers 1999). This means that it can take them longer to put the 'c' with the 'a' and the 't', and it might take them longer to say the word 'cat' if shown a picture of one. This can sometimes be linked to difficulties in what is referred to as 'working memory' or processing.

It is well established that children with DMD often struggle to develop phonological skills and have significantly more difficulties in learning to read than their peers and siblings (Billard *et al.* 1998; Hendriksen and Vles 2006). A recent Italian pilot study comparing dyslexia with DMD showed that both children with DMD and those with dyslexia showed specific difficulties in reading and writing words and in the time they took to name pictures on a page. Furthermore, the boys with DMD struggled with phonological processing in the same way as dyslexic children who had experienced a previous language delay (Astrea *et al.* 2015).

What is working memory and why is it important for reading?

This is the sort of short-term memory that we use to perform a particular task, for example, holding a number in our head while we take another number away from it, or holding a letter in our head while we place another letter next to it. Longitudinal research with younger children in the UK has suggested that the working memory skills of children as they begin formal education is a more powerful predictor of success six years later than IQ (Alloway and Alloway 2010). Working memory is a key skill needed in learning to both read and attempt arithmetic. This may seem like bad news for young people with DMD who have both established working memory and short-term memory difficulties (Hinton *et al.* 2007). However, even though we may never actually change a person's working memory ability *per se*, we can offer strategies to help them overcome these difficulties, in particular in areas such as reading and maths (look to the end of this chapter for ideas that support memory difficulties in these areas).

How helpful is IQ?

The vast majority of papers published about DMD and learning tend to focus on IQ. IQ stands for Intelligence Quotient and refers to a person's underlying ability, suggesting a concept of 'pure intelligence'. There are many reasons to have reservations about the use of IQ tests for any child, from their cultural bias, to the misleading suggestion that intelligence is something static (Gould 1981; Kamin 1977). Often due to the range of strengths and difficulties that children with DMD experience, a single IQ score can be quite meaningless. It is usually more helpful to look at the various sub-test scores in order to design appropriate intervention programmes.

As has been discussed in Chapters 1 and 2, a meta-analysis that looked at four decades of published studies found the average IQ to be lower in children with DMD than those without it, even though the majority did have scores in the average range (Cotton, Voudouris and Greenwood 2001). In a further analysis, Cotton and colleagues showed that the younger children scored significantly lower in the verbal tests than the older boys, suggesting that children with DMD experience specific language delay that can improve with age. The authors noted that the difficulties experienced by the younger boys in sub-tests such as arithmetic and coding were similar to those experienced by children with dyslexia or specific language impairment (Cotton, Voudouris and Greenwood 2005). Interestingly, in an earlier study where tests of arithmetic and digit span (working memory) were excluded, children with DMD did not gain a significantly lower IQ score than the control group (Whelan 1987).

The use of IQ scores can have far reaching effects. Over fifty years ago, researchers suggested that children with DMD were 'achieving within the average expectancy for children of their mental ability'

(Worden and Vignos 1962, p.971). Of course, if a young person with DMD does have more severe learning difficulties it may not be appropriate to enter them for a range of formal qualifications, or expect them to cope in a mainstream setting, and they may benefit from a variety of therapeutic interventions. However, if their low scores are due to specific difficulties associated with working memory or organising information, then it should be possible to offer relevant adjustments and appropriate intervention, as you would for someone with any other specific impairment like dyslexia, to ensure they achieve their potential.

In my experience of working with children and young people with DMD, it can often be easy to underestimate their abilities, because their difficulties can be more apparent than their strengths and they often struggle to communicate what they know. This can often lead to a child being moved to a specialist setting when in fact with the appropriate support and high expectations he could have achieved well in a mainstream school. Therefore any assessment must be accompanied by observations and conversations with the young person and their family.

Although IQ tests may not be particularly helpful in developing interventions they are still used in clinics and schools today, particularly if you are applying for an Education Health and Care Plan, so it is important to understand what they mean.

Understanding assessment scores

When a child undergoes a neuropsychological assessment he will complete many tests that have been standardised. This means they have been attempted by hundreds or even thousands of other children and young people of the same age in order to establish an average score for each age group. Therefore a standardised score will tell you how your child has performed in relation to other children of the same age. The 'average range' is anything between a standardised score of 85 and 115. In England, in order to qualify for 'access arrangements', which can provide extra time or a reader or scribe in formal examinations such as SATS or GCSEs, a child must score below a standardised score of 85 in tests for literacy or phonological processing. Standardised scores are converted into percentile ranks and these tell you how your child has performed in relation to 99 other children of the same age.

So if your child scored on the 99th percentile, only one child his age would have outperformed him; if he scored on the fifth percentile, 95 children of the same age would have done better than him.

Don't forget to look for strengths!

Hinton and colleagues assessed boys with DMD with a wide range of ability, and interestingly showed that, regardless of their IQ, they all showed a similar pattern in their strengths and difficulties (Hinton *et al.* 2000). In tests that required attention to complex verbal information such as digit span (working memory), comprehension and story memory, they all struggled, whereas on tests that demanded verbal understanding and abstract thinking skills they were able to articulate well-formulated responses. Tests like the British Picture Vocabulary Scale (BPVS) in the UK (The Peabody Test in the US) are helpful to show these strengths, and teachers are often surprised to find out how well a young person with DMD can score at this and how much they know. This is important when we are considering starting points for intervention as a child could well be more knowledgeable than he appears. If we can play to a child's strengths not only is he more confident and willing to attempt activities, but he is also more engaged.

The teaching of reading in schools

In England, the teaching of reading in schools has been influenced by Jim Rose's Review of Literacy Teaching (2009), which advises the adoption of the 'Simple View of Reading' (Gough and Tunmer 1986) as a framework for literacy development. The Simple View argues that reading is about getting meaning from the text, and without any meaning there is no reading. This model consists of two aspects – the ability to decode the text, and the ability to understand language.

When they start school most children have much better linguistic understanding than they do decoding skills. For example, they may know about dinosaurs or volcanoes but could not read or spell the words. Therefore, the focus given in early literacy classes is to develop the ability to decode so that children can access words that ultimately match their linguistic ability.

These decoding skills are now taught through the use of synthetic phonics. This means learning the 44 sounds of the phonetic alphabet and their corresponding written letters. Children learn that single sounds (or phonemes) can have one written letter (for example, 'a'), two written letters ('ea'), three written letters ('igh') or even four ('eigh'). These sounds are taught in a structured and systematic programme that enables children to match letters to sounds and ultimately blend these sounds together to make words (Rose 2009). Research in reading difficulties in both the UK and the US has shown the importance of phonological input that is in 'short bursts', that is, systematically organised in regular slots rather than one-off weekly sessions (Brooks 2007; Torgeson 2006).

As children with DMD are at risk of struggling to develop these decoding skills, the opportunity for 'over-learning' is important to make it an automatic process. This could mean extra individualised sessions to develop confidence in phonological skills necessary for reading, such as grapheme-phoneme correspondence and blending and segmenting words. If parents or teachers feel that the child is struggling to learn their sounds or blend them together, it is important to put in place a systematic programme that offers a multi-sensory approach so that the child can 'hear it, say it, see it and write it' (Reid 2016, p.166).

If you notice a child is struggling in these areas, do not wait for an assessment and diagnosis of dyslexia before you put any of this in place. A systematic, highly structured programme of study designed and monitored by a literacy specialist is important. For home, a pack of letter sounds and a small whiteboard with a dry-wipe pen can be a good starting place.

A starting point for reading intervention

Many remedial programmes focus on the areas where the child needs most help, but this can often mean him being presented over and over again with phonic tasks at which he will perceive himself failing. Where a child with DMD may have clear strengths as shown in their BPVS or Peabody scores, it can be helpful to place these phonic activities within a context of knowledge-based learning such as humanities, stories or social science subjects, while simultaneously working on areas of weakness such as the manipulation of sounds. It is important to stress that these strengths are relative to their other abilities, and may still be below the average score of their peers. This approach can help to alleviate the child's anxiety about learning and heightened feelings of failure, as well as further develop his vocabulary and knowledge.

The Decipha Programme

The Decipha Programme is an example of an approach that brings together the relative strengths of young people with DMD with what is known about best practice early reading intervention. The programme was developed as part of Action Duchenne's 'Include Duchenne' project which ran from 2008 to 2011 and worked with over 60 children, their families and schools across the UK. It was an online systematic and structured phonics programme, set in the context of time travel and delivered through a partnership between home and school over the course of one academic year. Parents led one 20-minute session per week at home, and a learning support assistant delivered four subsequent 20-minute sessions throughout the week at school. Children became 'time agents' travelling through different historical eras meeting ancient Egyptians, running away from dinosaurs in China, watching Vesuvius erupt in Italy and sitting next to Rosa Parks on the bus in Montgomery in 1955 to name just 4 of the 13 destinations. It has been suggested that vocabulary and knowledge can decrease in children with reading difficulties as they grow older and are not able to access age-appropriate books (Stanovich 1986) and so the opportunity for new learning experiences is important.

The results from the formalised evaluation of Decipha showed significant improvement in single word and text level reading, reading speed and comprehension (Hoskin and Fawcett 2014). Parent and school qualitative data were also positive. Several parents reported how challenging their children's behaviour could be, and how having a set time to sit down and look at a topic such as the Egyptians allowed them to see their children 'in a new light'. They reported surprise at how much their children knew about history and how engaged they were with the knowledge-based elements of the programme.

Developing reading fluency

As well as strategies for approaching words through phonics, learning high frequency whole words can be helpful (Ehri 1995) to develop fluency and make sense of the sentence. Paired reading can also help to support this. Paired reading is when an adult reads a sentence out loud themselves first, then reads it with the child and finally lets the child read it on their own. It is very important that the child is given any word they struggle to read, so that they can make sense of the sentence. The focus here is on fluency and not on phonic decoding.

Difficulties with writing

If a child has not developed the motor control to hold a pencil or form letters, using a finger from the writing hand to create letters in sand or paint, stirring cake mixture or writing in the air can all be helpful to support the development of early writing skills. A referral to an occupational therapist (OT) can offer specialist support in this area. Often problems with learning to write are connected to cognitive differences concerned with the development of automatic skills, rather than muscle problems (Nicolson *et al.* 2001). However, as the child gets older, writing can cause his hand to ache and thinking about alternative ways to capture text is important. This could include using a scribe or voice activated software, particularly if the young person has an extended piece of writing to produce. Many young people with DMD struggle to get started on a written piece, and the use of writing frames or scaffolds can be very beneficial, as can the use of mind maps to plan out questions in detail before starting them.

Issues with maths

Many children with DMD struggle with maths, and scores in arithmetic are often the lowest of all tests. There are a number of reasons for this, such as the working memory difficulties affecting the ability to perform calculations in your head, or accessing the words in mathematical word problems due to processing difficulties. Many younger children struggle to gain one to one correspondence when counting and to gain the automatic skills needed for doing simple addition and subtraction. General guidelines for those struggling with maths recommend making learning as concrete as possible. This is helpful, but at some point learning maths needs to become abstract. Often learning 'rules' can be helpful for some boys with DMD, but this is often contrary to current thinking that encourages children to understand the concepts. It is important as teachers and parents that we are flexible enough to try approaches that may not always be mainstream and which can play to any strengths a child may have, such as long-term memory.

Conversations and social communication

Holding conversations in fast moving situations with your friends or in a classroom at school requires concentration, focus and in a split second finding the right phrase or word to respond.

Impairments in phonological processing and working memory will affect this conversational process that most of us learn without much effort. Not being able to find the right word or phrase quickly and clearly can have a very significant effect on social relationships and self esteem. The result can be boys struggling to engage in conversations to the extent that they can get angry and frustrated about not being listened to or simply switch off. Friendships, joining in games, being 'one of the gang' all rely upon these fast and subtle social interactions. In addition, understanding social norms and cues can be a challenge for boys with DMD, which can sometimes mean they can appear odd or overbearing.

In a similar way, children with DMD can find it very difficult to process long strings of tasks or commands. Sometimes, it can seem that they are simply ignoring instructions when in fact they haven't processed them properly. It is important that boys are given time to respond in conversations and if necessary to learn with peers how to better manage conversations. These skills might need specific one to one or small group interventions where children are given opportunities to practice turn taking and listening.

Developing friendships

Some children with DMD who have social communication difficulties with perhaps a diagnosis of autism may find it more difficult to make friends. Moreover, some may lack a social smile and appear unfriendly and slightly eccentric. There are varied interventions that have been suggested for young people with social communication differences to help achieve inclusion. For example, Circle of Friends establishes a group of peers who fulfil a supporting role for the young person in question. This can be helpful when the child is younger and children are keen to help each other, and research has shown that it mainly serves to promote inclusion and empathy from classmates, rather than teach new skills to the young person with social communication difficulties (Frederickson and Turner 2003).

As teachers we often think if we get children to join clubs after school or at lunchtime then this can solve any friendship difficulties. With children who experience social communication differences this is often not enough. Of course it is important to find things that interest them and offer social opportunities, for example, Dr Who or Star Wars club might offer some children with DMD the chance to share expertise that is often hidden. However, just putting children together in a room to talk about their favourite subject does not mean they will develop the skills to communicate effectively and make friends. This is something that will require skillful facilitation and often prompting by adults and ideally be offered in partnership with some one to one skill development or coaching (see Chapter 5 for expert advice on this).

Similarly, it is important to offer opportunities at home to develop these skills. Play dates with other children can be helpful to support friendships and shared interests. Sometimes talking to other parents about DMD can help to give you as a parent a sense of control. This can be done in a variety of ways such as organising awareness-raising days or fundraisers. The importance of talking to your child and other children about DMD is discussed in Chapter 6.

Developing meta-cognitive skills

Helping a young person to understand how they learn best is very important. Even at a young age, children can discriminate between tasks they find easier and what they find more challenging. Using ideas taken from Solution Focused Brief Therapy (SFBT) and Collaborative Problem Solving, the young person can be supported to identify problem areas and to work out possible solutions (de Shazer and Dolan 2007; Green 2014). This can be a very helpful process for two reasons:

- It helps the child's ability to problem solve which is something many young people who have high anxiety or are inflexible struggle with.

- It means that the child is invested in any solutions that are put in place because they were his idea. This means they are more likely to work.

Solution Focused conversations are those which support the young person to focus on solutions, rather than on the current problem. So if a child identifies his desire to be a good reader or to have friends, he needs to be supported first to think about what that would actually look like, and second to identify what would need to be put in place to help that happen. SFBT focuses on what works rather than what doesn't, and supports the child to reflect on occasions when they felt things were working and how they could replicate this in the future. For more in depth discussion of and support with these methods, see Chapter 5.

Thinking about teaching assistants

Many boys with DMD who are at mainstream school are given one to one teaching assistants (TAs) to support them in the classroom. These support staff are often amazing at understanding and relating to our children and can almost become one of the family. However, it is important to take time to think about what the TA is actually there to do.

A six-year longitudinal study on TAs was published in 2009 which looked at the impact TAs had on the learning of 8,200 pupils in 78 primary and 92 secondary mainstream schools in England and Wales (Blatchford *et al.* 2009). This study found that the more support a pupil received from a TA, the less academic progress they made over a school year (consistent across years 1–10 and in all three core subjects).

This may seem very surprising considering the fantastic work we often see happening in school, and the energy we as parents have put into fighting for TA support for our sons. The researchers concluded that this was due to several reasons, none of which meant that TAs themselves were to blame, but rather were a result of the way the school or class teacher was deploying them. The most important finding was that young people with the most challenging difficulties were often getting very little input from the most qualified adult in the classroom, that is, the teacher. A further study by the same team looking at children with statements of special needs (old versions of Education Health and Care Plans) found that these children spent the equivalent of one day per week out of the classroom with a TA and away from the teacher and their peers (Webster and Blatchford 2013) and so had very little interaction with the teacher compared to children who did not have Special Educational Needs and Disabilities (SEND).

Additionally, research in the U.S. has warned that 'learned helplessness' can be an unintended consequence of high level TA support (Giangreco 2010). This often means that children come to depend on their TA to make decisions and spoonfeed them all of the answers, removing the need to engage in the task and in some cases even having the tasks completed for them! Having a TA 'velcroed' to a child in this way is not helpful and means that the child does not develop the ability to problem solve or become an independent learner. It can also deny the child the ability to learn how to get along with peers.

As a teacher it is important that you understand the learning and behaviour needs of the young person with DMD in your class and that you are actively involved in the planning, monitoring and assessment of his ongoing learning, even if it is the TA who will support him more closely.

If you are a TA it is crucial that you are given time to plan with the teacher and offered the training to help you give effective support. In her book for teaching assistants, Paula Bosanquet argues that TAs need to 'scaffold' the learning of young people with additional needs; supporting them to move forward into what was termed by Vygotsky as 'the zone of proximal development', in other words the place that they don't feel completely comfortable but where they are challenged enough to learn. (Bosanquet, Radford and Webster 2016; Vygotsky 1978)

As a parent you need to ask what any TA support is trying to achieve. As you will read about in Chapter 7, since the SEND Reforms in 2014, all resources and support should be linked to the outcomes you have co-produced on the Education Health and Care Plan. If you are worried that your child is not reaching these outcomes talk to school and find out what they are doing to help your child and how they are supporting the TA.

Checklist to support your child

1. Get an assessment

Always ask school to refer your child for a neuropsychological assessment if your child is starting school. In the UK this will usually mean a referral to an educational psychologist for learning areas and a clinical psychologist for social, emotional and behavioural issues. This will give you a fuller picture of how your child is doing and identify strengths and weaknesses, which is helpful when you are planning intervention. As a parent or teacher, ask if you can talk to the psychologist who is conducting the assessment so that they can explain the tests your child found easiest and most challenging.

2. Referral to outside agencies

Consider the input from specialists such as speech and language therapists and occupational therapists. Both can devise and monitor a programme for staff at school to implement, which can support articulation, language, social communication or the development of fine motor skills respectively.

3. Develop a home–school partnership to support reading

All schools in England should be following a programme of synthetic phonics. If you are a parent, ask school which reading programme they use so that you can support your child at home to learn these. As well as following a structured and systematic phonics programme, children need the chance to learn by reading whole words and sentences. This can be achieved through learning high frequency words and doing paired reading both at school and home.

If your child is struggling to read at the level of his peers, find other ways to help him access the same stories – for example, by either reading to him or through listening to story podcasts in bed. This means he is continuing to develop and access age-appropriate language and vocabulary even if he is unable to read it himself.

4. Support for working memory

If a child has working memory difficulties, think about breaking down instructions into chunks. Ask the child to tell you what he thinks he has been asked to do if you think he is struggling with processing language or short-term memory. Visual reminders around the classroom or by the front door can be helpful; for example, Have you remembered your book bag? Have you brushed your teeth? Sometimes, recording what someone says and playing it back can be helpful. If he struggles with visual short-term memory try and think of adjustments that don't mean lots of copying from the board – maybe handouts to stick in his book. Deliberate practice in phonics and/or numeracy that is short, structured and regular and that pushes a child outside his comfort zone, so that he is not just revisiting what he knows, is most helpful for skill development.

5. Look for strengths and interests

Find out what it is that your child with DMD is passionate about. This can sometimes mean hours of Star Wars conversations (!), but it's often important to enter his world to support his learning, rather than forcing him to enter yours. This can act as a starting point for any intervention.

6. Things to do at home

Support any preschool (and older) children with developing language – listen to songs, recite nursery rhymes and look at story books together. Have conversations about your day around the tea table and invite everyone to take turns and listen to each other.

Get out of the house – go to museums, galleries and anywhere of interest. Think about how to make learning fun and how you can support your child's interest in and excitement with the world. Have a go at board games. WARNING: This can sometimes be more effort than it is worth, as some children hate to play these. Others thrive.

7. Don't beat yourself up

As parents and teachers we tend to dwell on what has gone wrong instead of what we're doing right. Try to focus on what works well and do more of it.

8. Have high expectations

As you will discover in Chapter 7, which is about Education Health and Care Plans, it is so important to have the highest expectations from the outset. Ask your young person what it is they want to do when they grow up and as you go through the Education Health and Care Plan process think about what it is professionals need to do to make this happen.

Chapter Five

BEHAVIOR SOLUTIONS IN DMD

James Poysky

Introduction

If you are reading this chapter, it is probably because you know, or are related to, someone with DMD who has behavior problems. If it is a good day, you may be telling yourself that you want to learn strategies to help him have more success in school, at home, with friends, with life. If it's a bad day, you may be wondering if you can take it anymore without losing your sanity! You may be even be reading this because you are expecting it to validate your belief that the child just needs more discipline and his parents give in too easily to his demands. In any of these situations, you are not alone. For the rest of us (including helpful, stressed or exhausted parents, grandparents and teachers), behavior problems are a challenging component of DMD that affect many families.

Here is a person who has all the challenges of progressive muscle weakness, but on top of that they have behavior problems that can make their life so much more difficult. But it goes beyond that. Research has shown that behavior problems that occur in DMD can be just as stressful for parents as the physical/medical problems, sometimes even more so (Nereo, Fee and Hinton 2003). They can significantly disrupt family activities, exhaust and frustrate parents and others who are trying to help, and interfere with academic and social development in ways that can directly affect the child's short- and long-term quality of life. However, unlike the dearth of options available for the physical symptoms of DMD, the behavioral and emotional symptoms of DMD can be addressed in a comprehensive and robust manner. Does that mean it will fix everything? Of course not, but most families can obtain at least some degree of improvement.

Behavior problems and why they occur

There is an increased risk for behavior problems in boys who have Duchenne muscular dystrophy (DMD). In this regard, not all boys who have DMD will have behavior problems, but behavior problems occur more frequently than for children who do not have DMD.

It can be easy to view these behavior problems as the result of inept or overly-indulgent parenting, the child's attempt to make up for the loss of control over their own lives (as a result of their condition), or purposeful manipulation of people and circumstances in order to get what they want. While these things may be true in some cases, explanations like these fail to take into account the role of brain functioning.

The dystrophin protein, which has been described as a shock-absorber or project manager in muscle cells, is also found in the brain. As previously discussed in Chapter 1, there are also smaller isoforms, 'mini versions' of the dystrophin protein, that are also usually found in the brain. Depending on a child's specific genetic mutation, they may also be missing these smaller versions as well. Although research is ongoing and there is still a lot that is not known, there is significant evidence that points to changes in brain structure and brain functioning when dystrophin is absent (Doorenweerd *et al.* 2014). Similarly, research studies (Banihani *et al.* 2015; Cotton, Crowe and Voudouris 1998; Hendriksen and Vles 2006; Hinton *et al.* 2000; Perumal, Rajeswaran and Nalini 2015) have demonstrated increased risk for weaknesses in certain cognitive skills, such as language development, short-term memory, and acquisition of academic skills (i.e. learning disorders). If a child is also missing one of the smaller isoforms (a version called Dp140), they have an even greater risk of problems in these areas – beyond the increased risk they already have because of the absent primary dystrophin protein.

Traditionally, theories about behavior problems have typically been based on the premise that negative behaviors are occurring because they are being reinforced. In other words, kids engage in a pattern of problematic behavior because it is working out for them (yes, I realize I am over-simplifying, but this is essentially what it boils down to).

However, the 'behavior reinforcement theory' breaks down when we see a child who has a pattern of behavior problems that they continue to engage in, *even though it isn't working for them*. They end up getting into trouble frequently, adults and peers are mad at them, they are not doing well in school, they are unhappy much of the time, etc. So why do they keep doing it? Advances in neuropsychology and cognitive science have resulted in a gradual shift in how we view children with these kinds of problems. In this regard, children with recurrent behavior problems are believed to have weaknesses in certain kinds of cognitive skills. There are any number of cognitive areas that can be lagging behind, and no two children are the same. Based on my experience, I have found that some of the more common areas include impulse control, cognitive flexibility, emotional regulation, delaying gratification, communication, making inferences, anticipating consequences, planning/sequencing, and self-motivation. The area of weakness may not be directly related to intelligence, and you can see very smart children who have significant deficits in these skills. When the child is in a circumstance/situation that places demands on their cognitive skills that exceed their actual ability, they are unable to effectively navigate it and end up engaging in problematic/non-functional behaviors. This is why they continue to make the same mistakes, rather than learn from their mistakes and adjust accordingly. When abnormal brain functioning contributes to behavior problems, we refer to them as neurobehavioral disorders.

There is an increased risk of neurobehavioral disorders in children who have DMD (Donders and Taneja 2009; Poysky 2007). This means that it is important to keep in mind that the child's behavior problems may be occurring, to a large extent, as a result of abnormal brain functioning. It's neurological. This is important to remember, because it helps us set appropriate expectations, and to view the goal of our interactions with him to be focused on helping him learn new skills and strategies that he can then use to function better in situations that are difficult for him. In other words, the goal is to work with him, and meet him where he is at, rather than trying to fight against his skill deficits, expecting that this will make things better.

Additional factors can also contribute to why a child with DMD is having behavior problems, and what seems obvious at first glance may not always be what is really causing the difficulty. For example, a child may be avoiding their work in class not because they are lazy, but for a variety of reasons, such as they have reading difficulties, they did not understand the directions, they found the task too challenging/difficult/overwhelming, or they were distracted. Weaknesses in short-term memory may make it difficult for them to follow more than one direction at a time. Emotional distress may be making them more reactive and easily overwhelmed. Although this is not an exhaustive list, the following areas are the things that are most likely to be an issue for boys with DMD.

ADHD

Boys with DMD are at increased risk for having attention-deficit/hyperactivity disorder (ADHD). There are different kinds of ADHD, and it may not always look like what people think of when they picture a child with ADHD. Given the physical limitations associated with DMD, hyperactivity (running around, climbing on things, always moving) may not occur. More common are problems with impulsivity, such as talking too much, blurting things out, acting too silly, being impatient, and having difficulty stopping what they are doing (even when told directly). In other words, they can have difficulty 'putting on the brakes', and there does not seem to be much of a 'filter' between thoughts that pop into their head and what comes out their mouth.

Children like this are often described as 'immature'. Problems with attention can also occur, but not always in the manner that people expect. In this regard, boys with DMD who have attention problems can usually pay *excellent* attention to topics or activities that they find interesting. In fact, they can be *overly* focused on these activities, and they can have difficulty transitioning away from them. However, they have much more difficulty getting started on, and sustaining attention/effort for, activities that are *not* fun, but which they have to do anyway. For example, some boys can play video games for hours, but homework time is painful for everyone. Distractibility, rushing through things, careless mistakes, procrastination/work-avoidance, disorganization, difficulty following directions, forgetfulness, day-dreaming, and dilly-dallying are all features of this as well. Parents report that they have to repeat themselves numerous times before the child follows through with requests (not because they are oppositional, but just to get them moving). They may have to give prompts for each step for activities that should be routine (like getting ready in the morning), or else they would not be completed. It is also important to note that some boys with ADHD have greater problems with hyperactivity/impulsivity, while some may have greater problems with inattention (and related features). Some boys with DMD have problems with both aspects.

Social understanding/communication

Boys with DMD can be more likely to have weaknesses in their social skills (Hinton *et al.* 2006). In this regard, they can have difficulty engaging in reciprocal (back-and-forth) conversations. They may not say much (or not respond to what someone else has said), make random/tangential comments, or talk about something they are interested in – but which is not a topic the other person is interested in.

Boys with DMD can also have difficulty 'reading others', such as taking another's perspective, making inferences about things not stated directly, and using/interpreting nonverbal communication (e.g. facial expressions, body language). They may also be overly concrete in how they interpret things, and may not be as good at understanding non-literal phrases (e.g. phrases of speech or sarcasm). Sometimes the above noted weaknesses are so pronounced that the person may qualify for a diagnosis of an autism spectrum disorder. However, there are a number of boys who have milder weaknesses that do not meet diagnostic criteria, but can still make social interactions more challenging. For example, some boys do not automatically smile or say thank you to someone who has greeted them or helped them, and this can be interpreted by others as rudeness or lack of respect. Some boys with DMD can also be more withdrawn in social situations, particularly in group scenarios, or with people they don't know well. In some cases this may be occurring because the above noted weaknesses have resulted in a history of negative reactions from others, causing the child to become avoidant of potentially stressful, discouraging situations.

Arguing and angry outbursts

Boys with DMD can also be more likely to be oppositional and argumentative. They may be more contrary and disagreeable, almost as if they automatically say 'No!', no matter how reasonable the request. They are more likely to be described as hard-headed and stubborn, and can get their mind very set on how they want or expect things to be. When it doesn't turn out this way, they get 'stuck' and can't move on or adjust accordingly. This cognitive rigidity results in them becoming more entrenched in their view of how things should be, and they become argumentative – even when it is irrational. These boys can also have problems controlling their emotional reactions, in that they become angry very quickly, and have difficulty calming themselves down when upset. For some, this can manifest as temper tantrums and angry meltdowns that can be quite dramatic.

Attempts to curtail their arguing and angry outbursts that use threats or punishment tend to escalate things and make their behavior worse. These children are believed to have neurologically-based deficits in their ability to be flexible in their thinking, generate solutions, inhibit their emotional reaction, and make decisions based on future events. They are more likely to live 'in the moment', despite the fact that this may make things more difficult for them in the future. This is the child who will act based on how they feel right now, not on how they might feel later.

■ EXAMPLE

You have told your son that this weekend he can buy the X-BOX game for which he has been saving his money for four months (a miracle in itself). On Saturday you go the store, and they are sold out. He starts arguing and says he is not leaving the store without the game. He becomes 'stuck' and cannot get past the expectation that he would be able to walk out of the store with the game system. You tell him how ridiculous he is being, and that he is just going to have to wait until next week when more are delivered to the store. He starts yelling and stomping his feet, and refuses to leave the store. You tell him that he needs to stop and act his age, or else you are going to take away his X-BOX for a month. The yelling gets louder, and now he is crying and rolling around on the floor of GameStop. You then threaten to throw away his favorite toys, ground him until he is 20, etc. You end up having to drag him out of the store kicking and screaming. Yes, the meltdown happened because he didn't get what he wanted. However, the meltdown happened even though it was out of your power to meet his expectation.

The meltdown didn't make it any more likely that he would get his game.

A more accurate way to describe it is that the meltdown happened because he was very rigid in his expectations, and could not adjust them when they were forced to change. Attempts to stop his behavior with threats or punishments only made him more upset. He was not able to step back and say to himself, 'I'm not happy right now, but if I keep doing this I'm going to be even MORE unhappy.'

Anxiety and depression

Similar to other people with chronic illnesses, boys with DMD are at increased risk for experiencing anxiety and depression. Everyone feels sad and discouraged sometimes, and this is actually a normal response to difficult situations. Depression is different, in that it is more pervasive (happens most of the time, for longer periods of time) and interferes with daily activities, relationships, and goals. Children with depression do not necessarily look sad in the traditional sense. Instead, they can become more negative/pessimistic, irritable and grouchy, emotionally reactive, sensitive (feelings hurt easily, crying more), and self-critical. They may also become less motivated to do things that they used to enjoy, which is even worse when it comes to things they don't enjoy. They may be more likely to give up and become discouraged when things become challenging. They can also demonstrate changes in their energy level, in that they are more lethargic or, conversely, restless and agitated. Research has shown that, for the most part, younger boys with DMD do not appear depressed and are not overly concerned about their medical condition (Nereo and Hinton 2003). However, there is also evidence to suggest that this can become more prevalent during adolescence (Fitzpatrick, Barry and Garvey 1986).

Children with anxiety can be more likely to be fearful and worry about things. However, they may not always voice their fears and worries. Instead, they may be more avoidant of certain situations, ask frequent questions about what is going to happen, and need frequent reassurance.

Boys with DMD may also be more likely to have anxiety that occurs in response to unexpected events. For example, when there is a change in routine or some unexpected happens, they are easily 'thrown off', agitated, and out of sorts. This can be linked to the cognitive inflexibility mentioned in the earlier section. Similarly, they can also be more particular in how things should be. Sometimes this can be excessive, to the point where the child has obsessive-compulsive disorder. Social anxiety can also be problematic, and makes children more shy, quiet, and socially withdrawn unless they are around family members or people they know well. They may use electronics as a means of avoiding people in social situations (e.g. looking at their phone instead of having to interact with others). Although every child is different, depression is often viewed as a reaction to difficult circumstances. Children can also have anxiety as a reaction to difficult circumstances; however, in large part, the anxiety that occurs in children with DMD is believed to have neurological underpinnings and is best characterized as a neurobehavioral disorder.

Getting an assessment

The reader is strongly encouraged to review previous chapters covering cognitive functioning in DMD. In addition, any child with DMD who is demonstrating recurrent behavior problems should undergo a comprehensive neuropsychological evaluation. This can help pinpoint any weaknesses or neurobehavioral disorders that are contributing to the child's problems, as well as provide helpful advice about moving forward. Consultation with other professionals who are familiar with DMD is also highly recommended when a child has behavior problems, such as occupational/physical therapists, school psychologists, counselors/therapists, and psychiatrists.

Developing a plan

It is unlikely that you will find one simple thing that will address a child's behavior problems. The proverbial 'silver bullet' is a rarity in real life, probably because of the multitude of factors that can affect, and be affected by, behavior. Following a comprehensive assessment, and (hopefully) better understanding of what is happening, I usually encourage families to develop a multi-layered, multi-pronged plan to try to make things better. In this context, my bias is to have a tendency to recommend being as proactive as possible. I tend to see many people who have put things off too long, and the problems have grown accordingly. I guess I would prefer to err on the side of doing too much, and then having to pull back, rather than doing too little and trying to play 'catch-up'. It should also be kept in mind that there is no 'once then done', static approach to behavioral interventions. Rather, behavior intervention plans should evolve and adjust based on how the child is responding, what is working, what isn't working, and so forth.

When it comes to developing a comprehensive plan to address behavior problems, there is no one-size-fits-all approach. The details of any particular plan are going to (obviously) depend on the individual child and their family. However, at a minimum, I usually recommend coming up with a plan for school and a plan for home. There may be a high degree of overlap and similarity, but not always.

School plans may involve Special Education services, accommodations, and/or more informal supports. Teachers, school psychologists, tutors, educational therapists, physiotherapists, counselors, case managers, teaching assistants or aides, and other support staff may be involved. It is common for a child with behavior problems to also have learning problems. However, the behavior problems may overshadow the learning problems, or difficulty with schoolwork may be viewed as an outcome of the behavior problems. Unfortunately, both aspects need to be addressed in order to obtain progress in either area.

Home plans may include psychotherapy for the child, consultation with parents regarding strategies that they can use at home, medication, social skills training, and educational interventions (e.g. tutoring). People involved may include psychologists, psychiatrists, behavioral consultants/counselors, educational specialists and coaches as well as friends and members of the local community.

Helpful strategies

Most of the advice described below will focus primarily on problems with compliance (following directions), arguing, and emotional or angry outbursts because they are the behavior problems most frequently reported by teachers and parents. Keep in mind that there is no one approach that will work with every child, all the time. However, over time you will become better at being able to predict which approach is most likely to work in a given situation.

Medication

Medication should be a consideration for children with neurobehavioral disorders. Appropriate treatment with medication can help 'normalize' some of the brain dysfunction that contributes to their behavior problems. Getting the neurology of their problems under better control can help make other interventions more effective. Stimulant medications are the most effective approach for the treatment of ADHD symptoms, including both attention problems and hyperactivity/impulsivity. There are also several non-stimulant medications approved for the treatment of ADHD. These do not tend to work as well, but can be an option for children who cannot take or tolerate stimulant medications. Selective serotonin reuptake inhibitors (SSRIs) are helpful in addressing symptoms of anxiety and/or depression. Medication can also be helpful for problems with arguing and angry outbursts. The most effective medicine for these problems can depend on whether or not there is underlying ADHD and/or anxiety. Of course, medicine should never be used as the sole approach to addressing behavior problems, and should be one part of a comprehensive plan, which may also include various therapies, educational supports and parent training. The child's medical status, including cardiac health, should always be taken into account when medications are being considered. Consideration should also be given to potential negative interactions with other medications, as well as side effects that can have greater implications for those with DMD (e.g. potential weight gain).

General advice

There is no simple formula, nor easy solution, when it comes to addressing the behavior problems that occur with DMD. However, the more strategies that you can fall back on and employ in any given situation, the better. Over time, with practice (and lots of errors), you will get better about knowing what to use, and when to use it. Before we get into that though, here are some general things to consider.

- *Stay calm* when interacting with a DMD boy who is having behavior problems. [Pause to take 5 minutes to laugh hysterically at this advice.] OK, I realize this is impossible. We are all human, and it seems that behavior problems happen most often when it is most inconvenient. We are running late, we are tired/hungry, we have 20 other things that we have to do. The problem is that once we become angry, we are not good at problem solving, we make bad choices, and we tend to escalate things and make them worse. With this in mind, try to stay as calm as you can. Tell yourself that if you can stay calm, you are much more likely to 'win' this scenario…I mean help the child have a successful outcome. Also, keep in mind that it is important for us to model to the child how we want them to act.

- *Prioritize what you want to target* when it comes to behavior problems. You can't change everything all at once, and if you try you will fail miserably. So rank-order what specific behaviors you want to change. Think about when they occur, or when they cause the most difficulty. Try to be as specific as possible, and avoid generalizations. You are more likely to have success if you are targeting specific behaviors that occur at specific times, rather than trying to change behavior in a broad manner (e.g. you are more likely to make homework time faster and easier than you are to make him patient all day). Pick the top one or two, and work toward changing those behaviors. In doing so, you have to let some other behaviors go *for the time being*.

- *Make sure that expectations for behavior are realistic* for that child. Nothing causes more frustration and resentment, on all sides, than expectations that cannot be met. As parents and teachers, we often set expectations based on what we think a boy that age *should* be able to do, rather than based on what the child in front of us is *capable* of doing. This often occurs as the result of either misunderstanding the child's capabilities, or because it causes the adult stress to think that the child will not be able to master that age-appropriate skill. On the other hand, it is not helpful for the child's development if we have *no* expectations and cater to their every whim. The challenge is finding the middle ground. We want to set our expectations in a manner that will push them out of their comfort zone a little and challenge them to grow, but we also want to make sure that the expectations can be achieved. We want to set them up for success as much as we can. If they are not meeting expectations on a regular basis, then maybe we need to adjust.

- In general, *be clear when communicating expectations* for behavior. In this regard, try to be as specific as you can when describing what you would like to happen. Do not assume that the child will make inferences or 'know what you meant' unless you say it in a very specific manner. Err on the side of being overly specific. Be very concrete and direct about exactly what they need to do, rather than focusing on what you don't want them to do. Also, keep it short and simple. If you are droning on for more than a sentence or two, you have lost them. Similarly, if there are more than one or two steps, you should plan on giving them each step, one at a time. It can also be helpful for the child if you explain things in a manner that clearly indicates when they will be done (i.e. they need a light at the end of the tunnel). Here are some examples of helpful vs. unhelpful communication:

  Vague: 'Please clean up your room.'

  How clean is clean? My version might be different than yours, and then we can argue about that difference all evening. That is, after I get to it in two weeks because you didn't say when it needed to happen or how long I could take...

  Better: 'Once this episode of *Doctor Who* is over, I need you to clean your room. That means put the books on the shelf and the dirty clothes in the clothes bin. Also, any LEGO bricks not picked up and put in their bucket will be donated to charity.

You need to be done by 8 p.m. if you want cake…errr, I mean a healthy non-dessert alternative' (that last part was for any physicians and dietitions who might be reading).

- *Give advance notice of transitions.* Many boys with DMD can have problems making quick transitions, particularly if they are engaged in an activity that they really like. Thus, if you walk into their room and tell them that they need to turn their game off right now because it is time to leave, you are more likely to have a meltdown on your hands. Sometimes it can help to start the wheels turning in advance, by giving them reminders in a 'countdown' manner. For example, 'OK, in 30 minutes we need to leave.' 'OK, in 20 minutes we need to turn off the game and leave.' Then the 10 minute warning, five minute, two minute, one minute, 30 seconds, 15 seconds, etc.

- Try to *be as positive and encouraging as you can.* Children with behavior problems tend to get a lot of negative messages from others. 'Don't do that!' 'Why can't you ever…' 'I can't believe I have to keep telling you this…' 'When are you going to grow up?!'. Repetitive messages of this sort tend to cause discouragement and resentment, because the child feels like other people are always waiting for them to mess up. In the long run it can negatively affect self esteem, and can contribute to depression. What it doesn't do is cause them to do better. It can be easy to fall into the mental trap of thinking that if we are very consistent in pointing out everything they do wrong, then one day the light bulb will turn on, they will 'get it', and do a 180° course-change in their behavior. I can tell you that it doesn't happen. It doesn't cause the neurological underpinnings of their behavior to 're-wire' themselves. Similarly, if most of our communication with them is negative, they start to tune it out. We sound like a broken record. However, if most of the time we are positive and encouraging, those times when we do need to give negative feedback, it will really stand out. In addition, if the child feels like most of the time we are on their side, they are going to be more inclined to want to make us happy anyway. If they feel like we are mean and negative, they will think, 'Why bother?'

Effective reward strategies

Reward strategies can be helpful for improving motivation, effort, and compliance. They are much less helpful when used to target behaviors that occur because of deficits in other cognitive skills (e.g. phonics, language comprehension, reading ability, emotional reactivity, cognitive flexibility). This kind of approach is also more likely to result in success when used to target a very specific behavior or situation. Conversely, there is less likely to be success when this approach is used to obtain broad behavioral changes and/or for extended periods of time. For example, it is easier to come up with a plan to make homework time faster and easier tonight. It is much more difficult to make behavior better at school all day for the entire week, or to make the child follow directions the first time whenever they are at home. It is important to also keep in mind that the more often you use a reward system, the less effective it tends to become. It loses its glam, bling, or wow factor. Also, it is important that we don't send the message that the child never has to do anything unless they get something for it. The last thing I want to do is make my child a spoiled monster with DMD...that's what grandparents are for! Thus, we have to be strategic in how we use reward strategies. I would recommend using this kind of approach for the top one or two problems that cause the most difficulty and disrupt daily activities the most.

There are two important components to every reward system, and they need to be developed correctly for a reward system to work. If you set up a reward system and it doesn't work, it is because there is a flaw in one or both components.

1. The expectation

It is important to include the child in the process of setting up the reward system, as much as possible. The more involved they are, the more invested they will be. The more they 'buy in to it', the more motivated they will be to see it through. This may require us to be flexible in what we agree to, and we may need to (slightly) adjust our expectations to better fit what the child wants in order to keep them involved. I would recommend having a meeting with the child, wherein you sit down and discuss what the plan will be. First, describe the behavior or situation that you would like to improve. Try to avoid being overly critical of the child, and use objective phrasing as much as possible. Acknowledge that it is difficult for everyone, and everyone would like it if there was more success.

Mean Daddy: 'We need to talk about homework time. You make it really hard, despite my benevolent and altruistic desire to help you have academic success, because you argue with me every time I tell you to get started. Despite my being supremely patient, you end up making me mad because I feel like you are wasting my time. Don't you realize that Sunday evening is my only time to watch yesterday's Arsenal match that resulted (yet again) in a draw against an inferior team?'

Parent-of-the-Year Daddy: 'Let's talk about homework time. It seems like it is really hard on everyone. We both end up getting upset and saying unpleasant things. I know it feels like it is really hard and overwhelming to you. I end up getting frustrated because I don't like being the mean parent and forcing you to do it. We both have other things that we would like do instead of arguing and fighting over it. Let's come up with a plan together that makes us both satisfied. What do you think?'

Second, working with the child, define what needs to happen. As much as possible, avoid simply dictating what should happen and then getting them to agree to it. Try to encourage them to contribute ideas, give you their feedback, etc. Although I already discussed expectations in the previous section (General advice), it bears repeating here. Expectations need to be specific. Super specific. So specific that you think that they are needlessly specific. If you are reviewing the plan with them and the child tells you to *stop talking* because *they get it,* you might be on the right track. Specific expectations allow for everyone to understand and agree on what needs to happen, when it needs to happen, for how long it needs to happen, etc. This also makes it easier to determine whether the expectation was met or not. Also, you want to make sure the expectation is realistic. Nothing will cause a reward system to fail faster than expectations that cannot be met. In contrast, we want to set them up for success. It is not unusual for children to agree to expectations that are unrealistic, so it is important for the adult to step back and be as objective as possible. At the same time, you also want expectations to be difficult enough to challenge the child a little, and push them out of their comfort zone…in a manageable way.

Expectations should be defined in terms of what the child needs to do *right now*; short-term, rather than potential long-term outcomes. Also, expectations that can be met relatively quickly tend to be more effective than expectations that have to be met over long periods of time. The younger the child, the faster they have to be able to get that reward in their hot little hand. The sooner the better, immediately even, if possible. As they grow older they may be more able to work up to bigger rewards over time. However, I have found that for many older children and adolescents with DMD, it is difficult for them to go two to three days without being able to get their reward. Longer than this and their motivation drops off rapidly. Similarly, it is also important to avoid all-or-nothing expectations. For example, this could be seen in a reward system that expects the child to meet an expectation every day during the week to earn a reward on the weekend. The problem is that if the child fails to meet the expectation on Tuesday, then there is no incentive for the rest of the week. When reward systems are implemented in class, daily feedback should be sent home so that success can be further encouraged and rewarded.

2. The reward

For a reward to be effective it has to be powerful enough to do two things. First, the reward has to make the child so excited about it that he doesn't forget what he is supposed to do. It has to be good enough to stay in mind, despite whatever else may be going on in the child's life or surroundings. Second, the reward has to be exciting and motivating enough to override any negative feelings that the child has about what he is supposed to do. This means that the reward has to be good! Not good in our mind, but as determined by the child. Gold stars and stickers on a chart probably won't cut it for long, if at all. Everyone has an internal scale in their mind that they use to weigh the potential benefits of something against its drawbacks, and kids are no different. Basically, you have to make it worth it to them, and it has to be good. In an ideal world this would include things that are free, but let's face it, it's usually going to cost you. Also, once the novelty of the reward has worn off, it loses its effectiveness. This means that you have to be ready to change things up. And don't take rewards away once they have been earned, as this tends to feel very unfair to the child and will quickly undermine motivation.

Examples

Here are some examples of reward systems, and their associated strengths and weaknesses:

Example 1: An 8-year-old boy demonstrates a lot of resistance and procrastination when his mother tells him that it is time to get started on homework. This escalates, to the point where he is yelling, rolling around in the floor, and crying. His mother tells him that she has a plan. If he has good behavior in the evening Monday through Friday, then on Saturday she will take him to see a movie.

Critique: Good luck, Sister! The expectation of 'good behavior' is vague, and it is probably unrealistic for this to happen every evening. Plus, if he makes a mistake there is no incentive to keep trying.

Example 2: An 8-year-old boy is not completing his work in class because he is talking too much or out of his seat wandering around class. His teacher meets with him and they discuss what has been happening. They come up with a plan to increase the amount of time he stays in his seat and raises his hand, or is to be called upon before talking. His teacher breaks down the school day into 30 minute segments. She gives him reminders at the start of each time segment, and feedback at the end of each time segment. For every segment that he can stay in his seat and raise his hand before talking, he earns a point. Every time he earns four points he gets to play games on the class computer for 10 minutes.

Critique: Good plan. The expectations are specific, and possibly realistic. If he doesn't get a point for a time segment, there is incentive to keep trying in the next segment. Class computer time may be a strong enough reward, but this may need to be improved (or further rewarded at home).

Example 3: A 15-year-old boy has not been doing homework or preparing for exams, and spends most of his time playing on his X-Box. His parents take away his X-Box and mobile phone until he brings his grades up. Despite the fact that this should make him work harder (in their minds), it doesn't. They are further surprised when their lectures about 'good work habits' and 'being responsible' don't seem to resonate with him. He has been providing them with constructive criticism in return, informing them about 'how stupid they are' and 'how much he hates them'.

Critique: Yikes. The expectation of bringing his grades up is very vague. Better expectations would have focused on what he needs to do on a daily basis, which subsequently leads to improved grades. Also, this approach is more focused on working to avoid punishment than working to earn rewards.

Example 4: Another 15-year-old boy has not been doing his homework or preparing for exams, and spends most of his time playing games, watching videos, and messaging people on his mobile phone. His parents meet with him to discuss their concerns about what has been happening. They agree to a plan that will allow him to earn use of his mobile phone. He is expected to write down assignments in his planner, bring home the correct materials, and complete his homework and/or study between 6p.m. and 8p.m. every day. If he does not have any homework, then he will read ahead or use that time to study in advance for upcoming tests. Each day he does this, he will be allowed to have his mobile phone the following day. If he does not meet expectations, he will not be able to use his mobile phone the next day, but can always try again for the following day.

Critique: Not perfect, but better. The expectations are more specific, and there is always a reason to keep trying. It is also more focused on earning a privilege, than on something being taken away. This way it is up to him whether or not he gets his phone, and the parents don't have to make an arbitrary decision. Yes, I know that it can be difficult to make sure he is writing everything down and not 'forgetting' about any studying or other work that he should be doing, but you get the point.

Surprise rewards and other options

It is important for kids to have a clear understanding of what they have to do to meet expectations and earn rewards. However, we also don't want them always calculating the bare minimum that they need to do in order to get by. This is where surprise rewards can help. This is when you spontaneously choose to reward a child for something they have done, even though you did not talk about it in advance.

Sometimes there are activities that are difficult for the child, but are not really at the very top of the list of problem areas. For these lesser things, you can sometimes utilize a 'work then play' approach. In other words, they need to follow your request before they get to engage in things they like. For example, 'You can turn on electronics as soon as you put your dirty dishes in the sink.' If they don't put them in the sink, that's fine…but they are making the choice to not have the privilege. This approach puts the responsibility on them.

Using punishment

Although there are some parents who are overly-permissive, most children who have behavior problems end up getting into trouble often. Unfortunately, this does not tend to have a dramatic impact on the behavior problems.

I usually recommend that people use punishment as infrequently as possible. Try to restrict its use to situations where a child has broken a major rule, with malicious intent. These are times when the child knew what they were doing was wrong, and did it anyway. Also, the rule that was broken was very serious, and at the very top of the list of things that can never be done. Although this may vary from family to family, it may include things like stealing, breaking someone else's toy because you are mad at them, hitting, and lying (this last one can be tricky because sometimes they forget that they did something, and really think they are being honest). In these kinds of situations, punishment should be used to send the message that their behavior is not acceptable under any circumstances. Probably not included on this list are things like not following directions, getting angry/arguing, being selfish, making a mess, breaking something because they were careless.

When punishment is warranted, it should be powerful but brief. By powerful, I am not referring to physical punishment like spanking. Rather, in whatever form it takes it should be viewed as very unpleasant by the child. It can be difficult to figure out what this should be, because the child will not necessarily let you know that they don't like it. You have to make your best choice and stick with it. Also, the punishment should be relatively brief. This allows the child a chance for redemption, a chance to try again. Don't get caught into an escalation cycle, where you keep escalating the level of punishment because the child keeps acting out or their behavior becomes even worse. Things tend to get blown way out of proportion, and whatever lesson we were originally trying to teach gets lost in the storm.

For rule violations that are not at the top of the list, maybe things we would call 'medium' violations, try to focus on teaching responsibility and making things right. The main point is less about 'you're in trouble', and more about 'you messed up, now take care of it'.

For example, several years ago my son used a permanent red pen to color on our neighbors' gutter downspout. I explained that he wasn't in trouble, but he was not allowed to do that because it was not our property, it ruined their paint, etc. I took him next door to apologize and we explained his mistake (honestly, this was probably more painful for him than any punishment I could have thought up, but that's not the point). Then we took some money he had saved, went to the hardware store, and bought some matching paint. Then we went back and painted it (which means that he stood next to me while I painted it). Then I was able to tell him how proud I was of him, and we moved on.

Not every situation lends itself to this kind of intervention, but we could probably use this approach more often than we do. Keep in mind that if you have a child who is neurologically predisposed to make a lot of mistakes, we are not likely to have success if we are sending them the message (by punishing them) that they cannot mess up. We are much more likely to have success as parents if instead we are trying to teach them that when they *do* mess up, they need to make it right.

Then we come to the minor things. The things that, in the big picture of life, are probably not that important. However, these are the things that happen frequently, and drive us mad. The interrupting, being too loud, not following through despite being asked 10 times, making messes, being rude, chewing with their mouth open, and on and on. These are the things that will keep happening no matter what you do. You can pick one or two of them to focus on, but you can't address all of them. Because of this, you need to accept that these are the things that we have to be patient with. We have to accept that we will have to repeat ourselves, do some things for them or else they will never get done, and ignore their annoying or immature behaviors. Don't get caught in the thought trap that if you are really consistent, and point out every mistake, and jump on every minor behavioral infraction, that one day the light bulb will turn on, they will see the pattern, and everything will get better. This doesn't happen. Instead, they end up getting in trouble all the time, hearing a lot of criticism, and feel like they can never make you happy no matter how hard they try.

De-escalating and problem solving

Some boys with DMD can have frequent problems with being argumentative and oppositional. They can be very rigid in how they expect things to be, and when it doesn't turn out that way they get 'stuck'. They can't move on, no matter how irrational or dysfunctional it may seem. If challenged or contradicted, they seem to become even more entrenched in their expectation. This often coincides with their tendency to become easily frustrated, and they can have subsequent angry, explosive outbursts. As previously mentioned, these behaviors can be related to weaknesses in specific cognitive processing and problem-solving skills. In particular, children like this appear to have a deficit in their ability to be adaptive in their thought process, or modify their views and generate new solutions in response to unexpected circumstances. When they are put into situations that place demands on their area of weakness, in a manner that exceeds their ability, they argue and explode. These children tend to live in the moment, and have more difficulty making decisions based on how they might feel in the future. This is why they tend to become more upset and escalate things when parents attempt to control their arguing and emotional outbursts with threats or punishment. In other words, trying to force them to be flexible often results in them becoming more rigid and stuck.

This is difficult to fight against, and an approach that is focused on teaching them who the boss is or 'breaking their stubbornness' rarely works with children like this. Instead, the goal should be to look for opportunities that can be used to teach new skills and better problem solving in a supportive, instead of antagonistic, manner. This means you may have to change how you look at the child's meltdowns and negative acting out. Don't view it as a situation in which your primary goal is to control their behavior and make it stop. Instead, view their arguing, oppositional behavior, or meltdown as a signal, in which they are telling you, 'I'm stuck!' This is important, because it helps us avoid getting caught in power struggles, prevents us from getting side-tracked by something less relevant, and keeps us focused on the underlying skill deficiency that is contributing to the negative behaviors.

For example, imagine a child starts pitching a fit and having a meltdown because you turned off his video game in the middle of him playing it (after you had asked him 10 times to turn it off). He begins yelling, crying, rolling around on the floor, and he tells you that you are a big, stupid, fart-face who smells like poo. You tell him that he is are not allowed to talk to you that way, you are in charge, and now you are going to take away video games for a month. He becomes more angry, tells you that he doesn't care because he hates you, and he throws your iPad at the wall as hard as he can. Your reaction is to tell him you are going to throw away all his toys, lock him in the dungeon, and make him eat broccoli for every meal. In response, he begins slamming all the doors as hard as he can, pulling everything off the bookshelf, throwing his shoes at the dog, and screaming at the top of his lungs for the neighbors to call the police because you are hurting him. (I'm not exaggerating, this is a real-life example.)

I call this scenario the 'Tornado of Terror'. Things quickly escalate far beyond whatever the original problem was, to the point where we lose sight of our initial intent. The above kind of parenting approach tends to be rooted in a parenting philosophy that believes our primary goal in that situation is to force compliance. To what I say, whether you like it or not. This includes both the turning off the game when I say so, but also for the child to not express his unhappiness in such a manner. The problem with this approach is that, even if it does force compliance on rare occasions, it does not address the underlying weaknesses that caused the child to act that way in the first place. Next time this situation rolls around again, we will be having the same battle.

Step 1: Changing your mindset

In order to help the child learn new skills, you have to change how you view your role as the adult. You are no longer the boss, who dictates what the child should say or do, the one who forces the child to act in a more mature manner because life is hard and if they don't learn to be responsible now their life will be ruined (yes, I'm exaggerating to make a point). You have to view your new role as primarily that of a coach, teammate, and teacher. You will have to avoid getting caught up in trying to control the behavior you see on the surface (arguing, talking back, yelling, etc.). Instead, you are going to try to focus on the underlying weakness that is causing the behavior. This means that you have to let some things slide in order to do so, and avoid getting side-tracked by responding to the child's behavior 'in the moment'. This means that instead of dropping the hammer down because he is crying, yelling, and arguing with you about turning off his game, you are going to utilize a different approach that will, hopefully in the long run, give him new, more functional ways of dealing with disagreements and frustration.

Don't misunderstand me: there will always be situations in which an adult has to send the message that what the child is doing is unacceptable and needs to stop. Using threats and punishment in these situations is sometimes warranted. But we want these kinds of situations to be few and far between, and use this kind of approach as infrequently as possible. As adults, we tend to resort to this kind of approach much more often than is really necessary. We also have to accept that if we decide that the child's current behavior absolutely *must* stop right now, no matter what, and I am going to implement a punishment in order to make it happen, then I also have to accept that he is probably going to have a meltdown and try to escalate things.

Step 2: Changing your communication (active listening)

If you see that a child is starting to send up signals that he is stuck and can't navigate a particular situation, your job is to try to connect with him socially and emotionally. You want to show him that, even if you disagree with him, you are on his side and want to try to help him figure things out. One of the most effective ways to demonstrate this is to use active listening skills. Everyone has heard of this term, but most people don't know what it really means. Well, to start off, let me tell you what it *isn't*.

It isn't listening to the child enough so that you can point out how they are wrong. 'I know you're mad about me turning off the game, but this is the consequence of choices you have made.'

It also isn't listening to what the child is saying, just so that you can step in and give them advice. 'I know you're mad, but next time you can listen to me the first time when I ask you to do something.'

It isn't minimizing the child's distress or frustration. 'Why are you so mad about this? It's not that big a deal!'

All of these things may be true, but when the child is stuck and starting to freak-out, meltdown or argue he is not going to be able to hear these things. At least, not yet.

Active listening is also, duh, not lecturing. I know it sounds obvious, but you'd be surprised at how often people do this when they think they are using active listening. So make sure you are being quiet when you are actively listening. Your goal is to get the child to start to learn how to better communicate what they are thinking and feeling. You also want to help them feel understood and accepted; it is a chance for empathy and emotional support. Basically, when they start freaking out, you want to talk it to death.

There are probably many different aspects of active listening, but here are some of the main ones:

- *Validate the child's feelings.* Acknowledge how they are feeling, and your understanding of why they feel this way. This also allows you to show that how they feel is important to you. You can do this *even if you disagree with them or don't think they should feel that way.* Of course, for this to work you have to be genuine in what you say. Sarcasm doesn't tend to fly that well ('Ooooh, you're mad *again*, I see!').

- *Ask open-ended questions.* These are questions that can't be answered with a yes/no or one-word answer. They encourage talking. What happened? What led up to this? What did you want to happen instead? What was the worst part of it? How has this compared to things like this in the past? Open-ended questions also allow the child to maintain control of where the conversation is heading. Our use of very specific or yes/no questions essentially results in us commandeering the conversation. This can actually cause us to miss something important that is going on. One additional word of advice, try to avoid asking, 'Why?' People perceive this to be judgmental. There are also open-ended phrases that aren't really questions, but can still encourage talking ('Tell me more.').

- *Paraphrase content/context.* Basically, describe what you see happening, what you are hearing. This is like summarizing what is going on. ('So, let me make sure I understand. You were in the middle of playing the game, and you were really excited because you'd just made it to a new level that had previously given you trouble. When I came in and shut off your game, you felt like it wasn't fair, and that I wasn't being sensitive to how important it was to you.')

Active listening is a skill that has to be fostered. I have training in this, and I am lucky if I can do it 15 percent of the time. My wife would probably say 5 percent. However, in as much as we can do it, it can really make a difference. I have found that if you can become marginally proficient in active listening and apply it in these meltdown/conflict situations, nine times out of 10 that is all you need to do. Crisis averted. Sometimes, once they have felt heard and accepted, and things have calmed down, children are much more open to hearing what you have to say (e.g. advice, pointing out their mistakes, telling them it wasn't that big a deal).

Step 3: Brainstorming

So, after things have calmed down and we have used our active listening skills as far as we can go, then it is time to promote problem solving. The goal is to communicate to the child, 'Hey, I am sure that together we can work this out and think of a solution that makes both of us satisfied.' You want to do it together, in a 'Let's-be-a-team-in-this' manner. You want to emphasize that *both* people need to be satisfied with the solution, not just you, and not just the child. Both people are important. Step 3 requires that, as the adult, you are going to need to be flexible in how you generate and adopt potential solutions. It requires compromise from both people. I know this might feel weird, but it goes back to what is the priority in that moment. Is your primary goal as the adult to teach the child that he has to do everything that others tell him, or is the primary goal to teach the child how to think of solutions and work toward compromise with others? In my mind, that latter is a much more valuable skill to have. When going through the brainstorming process, it can be tempting to be the one to generate all the ideas. However, we really want the child to start to be able to do this, so try to have him think of at least one idea. Initially, all of the 'solutions' that the child generates will be totally unrealistic, or will be completely slanted in his favour. Keep referring back to needing to make everyone satisfied. If he starts arguing or getting worked up, revert back to your active listening mode. Over time you will find that he will get better in thinking of more realistic, balanced ideas.

Step 4: Try it out and adjust as needed

When you both agree on a potential solution, try it out and see how it goes. Initially most of the solutions you pick will not end up working out. This can be for a variety of reasons, such as the child agreed to something they could not follow through with, there was some other problem that we weren't aware of that was contributing to the initial problem, etc. However, it's OK if the solution you pick doesn't work out, because the primary goal is learning the *process*. If one didn't work out, you remember and take it into account the next time a similar solution pops up. ('Remember when we tried that last time, and it didn't work out? How can we do it different this time so that it will work better?')

Keep in mind that, in the same way it takes the adult a while to get good at this process, it also takes some practice on the part of the child for them to know their role. Initially, they may be a little suspicious. What is mom up to? Why isn't she yelling at me and sending me to my room? At some point he may even start to realize what you are doing, and will try to sabotage it on purpose. A few years back I was doing this with my son and he told me, 'Don't do that doctor crap with me!' Stick with it, because even then it still works. Eventually he will realize that you have good intentions, and that it actually makes things work out better. He is less angry, less often in trouble, and feels like the two of you are having more positive interactions.

Please note that I am not smart enough to come up with the above noted strategies on my own. For more information from the real sources, please refer to books covering 'Emotion Coaching' (The Gottman Institute 2017) and 'Collaborative Problem Solving' (Lives in the Balance 2017).

Chapter Six

TALKING TO CHILDREN ABOUT DUCHENNE MUSCULAR DYSTROPHY

David Schonfeld

Informing children of their diagnosis and starting the discussion

Generally, the best time to inform children that they have DMD is soon after it first becomes known. Parents' inclinations may be quite different. They may want to shield their children from learning difficult news about their health. Parents may think it best to wait until children are 'ready' to accept the information, or at least until they themselves have come to terms with the diagnosis and its implications. Parents may justify the delay by questioning if their children are even ready yet to understand what it all means. They may decide to wait until the 'right time' to tell their children, or at least until a better time. The task may seem so overwhelming that they simply decide to put it off until later.

While it is understandable that parents want their children to believe they are safe and healthy, the reality is that children can tell when parents and other close relatives in their lives are worried or upset. Even if they haven't been told anything, children sense that something is wrong. Knowing that something is wrong and having no idea what it is can be unsettling even for young children. When parents decide to withhold information from their children, the adults that are aware have to devote a lot of time and energy to maintain secrecy – at a time when they have little of both. It limits the adults' ability to readily access information and to provide support to each other and of course makes it impossible to provide any such support to the children. Chances are that children will find out inadvertently, such as by overhearing comments (e.g. a nutritionist that comments during a clinic visit the importance of watching the child's weight gain because otherwise he will be too heavy to lift out of his wheelchair when he gets older). When children only get piecemeal information about their medical condition it's likely that their understanding will be limited; they may have major gaps in their comprehension and significant misunderstandings (e.g. I ate another cookie when my mum wasn't looking – will that mean I may not be able to walk in the morning?). Learning about DMD from overhearing a comment or figuring it out on their own is not the best way for children to first learn of their condition.

Misleading children, even when the motivation is entirely well-intentioned, may erode children's trust and lead to anger and withdrawal. It may communicate to children that their parents are not willing or able to answer questions, provide information, or offer support. The current expectation for children with DMD is eventual progression of illness which requires an increasing dependence on adult caregivers – often the parents. Such dependence should have a firm foundation of trust and mutual respect.

It's true that very young children can't easily understand much about DMD – at least not at first. But the only way they will ultimately understand is to be taught and the sooner the process is started, the sooner progress is made. We explain to children that we need to put the milk in the refrigerator when they are very young – before they know how to pronounce 'refrigerator' and certainly well before they understand the mechanism of coolants or the science behind why milk spoils at warmer temperatures. They would never understand all of this unless we started to explain what a refrigerator was at a young age. They grow into their understanding.

A 5-year-old might first be told that he has Duchenne muscular dystrophy – or Duchenne's (or DMD) for short – and given an explanation such as the following:

> Duchenne is a medical condition that some children are born with that makes their muscles weaker. That's why you sometimes trip when

you run or have sore legs at the end of the day. It isn't an illness, like a cold, that can be spread to other people; you don't get the illness because you did anything wrong. Duchenne is the name of the person that first described the illness and 'muscular dystrophy' means that the muscles don't work as well. It bothers us that you have this illness because the doctors don't yet know how to cure it – which means to make it better and not have it come back. But fortunately, there are medicines you can take and exercises you can do to keep your muscles as healthy as possible for as long as possible. We will work with your doctor and the team at the clinic to keep your muscles as strong as possible.

Then pause for questions. Don't be surprised if children don't get it all the first time, or if they ask some of the same questions more than once. As time passes and they develop a better understanding of illness in general, as well as accumulate more information about DMD, they may ask the same questions again or ask entirely new ones. Focus your discussion on practical information that is relevant presently or likely to be important in the near future. Don't focus on long-term prognosis – young children tend to be most concerned about what impacts them now. Besides, chances are the prognosis will improve in the future.

If you start the conversation about DMD when children are very young, it's easier for everyone. At young ages, children often don't have many or even any symptoms and aren't likely to be aware of or interested in long-term outcomes associated with the illness. Parents don't have a lot to explain at first and what children need to understand is more balanced with their capacity to understand. It's similar to introducing the topic of sexuality with children. If you start when children are toddlers by introducing the names of body parts, and then explain what those body parts are for in simple terms during the preschool period, it's not overwhelming for children or their parents. But parents who wait until their children's wedding night to have their first conversation on the topic are likely to be met with a very awkward (and most likely moot) discussion. And these children are unlikely to turn to their parents in the future when they have questions on this topic or related problems for which they want help. They are also less likely to turn to their parents when they have important questions or problems even in unrelated areas.

Parents may be tempted to wait to first talk with their children until they, themselves, are coping well with the diagnosis and its implications. People often reference the airline safety presentation where adults are instructed to secure the oxygen mask on themselves first, before helping their children. While this is good and relevant advice and does serve as an important metaphor, there is a limit to how long you can wait until helping children. Some airlines have added a clock to the printed instructions to clarify that you need to help your children with their mask within two to three seconds. You can't wait until you are comfortable with the fact that the oxygen level in the cabin has dropped before you address your children's needs – you may never be comfortable with that reality. The same is true with DMD. While it is appropriate for parents to be told about their son's condition before the children are informed, the delay in telling the children themselves should be very brief.

That means that parents will be talking with children before they know a great deal about DMD and most importantly, before they feel comfortable talking about it. But parents only need to know enough about DMD to begin the conversation and answer the early questions. If there's a particular question for which parents don't know the answer, such as whether dogs get DMD like people do (yes, there is an animal model of DMD involving dogs), they can promise to look into it and return with the information. For older children, parents can look for the answer to some of these questions together and help children figure out where and how to get accurate information on the internet.

Although children may have more experience and comfort finding information on the internet than their parents do, children may have less knowledge of how to determine the accuracy and appropriateness of what they find on the internet. While we want children to turn to their parents, other adults in the family, and the healthcare team as the primary sources of information about their medical condition and its treatment, we need to recognize that children (and adults) are likely to turn to the internet to answer some of their questions or to try to confirm what they were told. So although you may suggest to children that they should ask you or the healthcare team when they have questions or would like more information about their illness or its treatment, you should make it clear that if they do learn of something from others or on the internet, they shouldn't hesitate to ask you or their healthcare team how to interpret that information and what it might mean specifically for them.

Information on the internet isn't tailored to the child's own condition. Information on long-term prognosis is based on follow-up of children treated many years ago who weren't able to benefit from the treatments your children are now receiving and certainly not the treatments that may be discovered or become available in the future. Not all children have the same severity of illness or experience the same complications. Information about outcomes, prognosis, or complications that is found on the internet may be hard to apply to an individual child – this is why the healthcare team that knows the information *and* knows the particular child and his condition is in the best position to help answer some of these questions.

For parents who already have waited months or years, so they no longer have the opportunity to tell their children soon after diagnosis, the next best option is tell them now. You can't go back in time to tell them earlier and there is no benefit in waiting further. If older children question why they weren't told earlier or show anger at being misled, parents can explain that they acted in what they thought was their children's best interest and wish they had started the conversation earlier.

Even parents who know their children well and benefit from a close relationship may not be aware of what children already know or suspect. Children learn from a young age when their questions about their health problems make adults uncomfortable and may avoid asking further questions so as not to upset them. They pick up on the cue that their parents don't want to discuss this or even to let them know and they may enter into a mutual pretense that they are unaware of their medical condition. But that doesn't mean that they are unaware. This silence does mean that children have to deal with their concerns alone, without support, and without adequate information, which is why it is important to begin the conversation.

How to explain illness and its treatment

Older children understand more about illness in general as well as about a specific medical condition, not simply because they have accumulated more factual information or been given more explanations.

There are also developmental changes in the way children interpret and understand the information that is provided to them. Adults should aim to provide explanations that are consistent with children's current understanding of illness and that aim to take them to the next level.

Very young children tend to rely on magical thinking and explanations that attribute the cause of illness to what has been called "immanent justice'. This is a belief that good is naturally rewarded and misdeeds, even if only contemplated, are punished. These immanent justice explanations can result in guilt and shame being associated with illness – and some of this remains well into adulthood. They may view their medical condition and its treatment as a punishment for something they did or considered doing, or something they failed to do. It's best to avoid the term 'bad' in talking about DMD (for example, 'DMD is a bad sickness') and to make sure you tell children directly they didn't get DMD because of anything they did or didn't do. We don't want children to see the treatments for DMD (whether that be medication that can cause undesired side effects or exercises that may be uncomfortable, inconvenient or painful) as punishments. Rather, they need to come to a basic understanding (that should become more sophisticated over time as their level of understanding of illness develops) of why they are being asked to accept these treatments. If children don't understand why and resent the treatments, they are more likely to resist them and noncompliance will increase. Adults, who may be frustrated by children's resistance to cooperate fully, may add to this when they use 'threats' of the need for increasing treatment, such as 'You may think these exercises hurt, but if you don't do your exercises regularly your muscles will get tight and then you'll need surgery – and that's going to hurt even more!' But then if surgery is required, children are more inclined to see it as their fault, even if it is the result of the natural progression of the illness despite full compliance with preventive measures. While immanent justice explanations are common among children, they are less likely to persist when children are given accurate information and helped to understand the cause of their illness. Given that these immanent justice explanations are often associated with feelings of guilt and shame, helping children develop a more accurate understanding of the cause of their illness is likely to promote their overall adjustment and ability to cope with the treatment process.

As children develop more of an understanding of their medical condition, adults should be looking for different potential areas of misunderstanding. This may be due to gaps in information (i.e. they assumed something because they weren't told the real reason – such as assuming you can spread DMD the same way you catch a cold, because they haven't heard that you get DMD differently), misinformation (e.g. they read something on the internet that was incorrect or misheard information in a conversation that they overheard), literal misinterpretation (i.e. they heard correct information but misinterpreted it – such as confusing 'passed out' with 'passed away' and concluding that a child that had fainted from a medical condition had instead died), or misconception (i.e. they applied inaccurate reasoning to come up with an incorrect understanding, such as a child that assumes because he is the oldest child in the pediatric DMD clinic that he is likely to die soon, not realizing that older adolescents are followed in a clinic at the adult hospital).

In order to minimize such misunderstandings, use simple and direct language – avoid jargon, unnecessary medical terminology, and extraneous details. For example, you shouldn't aim for children to understand diagnostic test results, but rather help them understand relevant implications – they don't need to be able to review their radiology studies, but they should be aware of what was learned from the procedure that is relevant to them, such as it shows that there hasn't been much new damage to their muscles since the last study. Focus your initial discussion on the immediate and near future – 'soon' for children may mean before dinner or bedtime, rather than sometime in the next five to 10 years.

Continuing the discussion

The amount of information to share with particular children depends not only on their age and developmental level, but also their coping style, and the extent to which they are anxious, obsessive, or have other characteristics that may make it difficult for them to cope with additional, or particular, types of information. Some people are better able to cope with a difficult situation when they understand more about it, whereas some children (and adults) may find additional information sensitizing. Consider starting with asking children what they already know or have heard and then provide basic information that is directly relevant to the children in simple and direct terms. Then ask them what questions they have and what further information they want. It is sometimes helpful after providing important and potentially complicated information to children to ask them to explain back what they have learned and follow-up with questions to probe their understanding. This may help you identify gaps in their information or comprehension, or misunderstandings or misconceptions that you can help correct.

Don't try to cover everything in one or even a couple conversations. The goal is to start a conversation that you plan to continue indefinitely. As children accumulate more experience and knowledge and as their cognitive development advances, they will likely come up with new questions. They may also return to the same questions you already answered before, either because the prior answers weren't satisfying or because now they want and are ready to develop a better understanding. Milestones in their life – whether due to loss of function (such as when they need to use a wheelchair to get around) which may be associated with additional adjustment difficulties or developmental achievements (such as high school graduation) may prompt new questions and new concerns. Sometimes the questions come from seemingly nowhere – a comment that was overheard, a question that was generated during a moment of reflection, a story or picture that triggered an association. Some questions are rhetorical (e.g. 'Why did I have to be the one to get this illness?!'); at times, children may be seeking support rather than answers. If the question comes up at a time when it is impractical to discuss (e.g. such as when you are dropping your son off at school while you are late for work), try to figure out if it is urgent to answer at that moment (it's usually not) – and if not, let your son know you will talk about it soon when you are both together again and able to talk. And then be sure to follow-up on that promise.

Helping children cope with their concerns about their illness

Parents should recognize that children may have very different concerns and worries than adults. So it's important that children are invited to share their specific concerns or questions. Some of their concerns may be the result of misunderstandings and limited or inaccurate information. But some of their worries may be based on realistic concerns. Try to avoid telling children they shouldn't be worried or concerned – even if you believe their particular concern isn't that bad or shouldn't be causing as much distress. Allow them to own their feelings. If they feel worried, they are worried. While you can certainly clarify why you are not as concerned, if they personally remain concerned, help them figure out how to cope with that worry.

While you don't want to dismiss their concerns or provide false reassurances, don't eliminate hope either. Children should feel that their lives are filled with potential – because they are even for children diagnosed with DMD. If a 5-year-old says he wants to be an astronaut, it's fine to tell them that that would be a really special job and ask why he wants to be an astronaut. Don't feel the need to explain that his diagnosis is going to make it very unlikely that he could travel to the moon. The reality is that it is very unlikely any other 5-year-old child is going to travel to the moon. Children should be allowed to have their dreams, even if they seem unrealistic, as long as they take the appropriate steps to do what they need to now in order to preserve their health, and comply with treatment regimens, and don't ignore developing other skills and pursuing other opportunities that are more likely to be achieved. As young people are living with DMD longer and able to lead more productive lives, it becomes increasingly important that children with DMD have career aspirations and are encouraged to strive for careers that are personally meaningful to them, yet achievable within likely constraints placed by their illness.

Parents are often reluctant to share their own concerns, worries, and troubling feelings with children. But while it isn't helpful for children to see their parents overwhelmed or devastated, it is helpful for children to hear some of your concerns or feelings and how you have successfully coped with them. This encourages them to share their worries and feelings and also gives them some ideas about coping strategies. Children can't learn how to cope with troubling feelings unless the adults they trust share some of their distress and model and teach them how to cope. As other members of the family share their own individual coping strategies (e.g. talking with others, journaling, expressive arts, exercise, progressive relaxation, mindfulness, providing service to others, etc.), children begin to build a toolkit of options they can choose from to use themselves.

Parents may also wish to consider consciously teaching coping strategies at a young age, even before they may seem required, so they can master the skills before they are most needed. For example, children can be taught self-hypnosis techniques that can be used to deal with pain and anxiety. Children with DMD are at higher likelihood to develop anxiety, and the progression of the disease and resulting worsening of motor skills or respiratory effort is likely to be anxiety provoking for anyone. How individuals adjust to a situation depends in large part on how they understand and interpret associated experiences. Cognitive behavioral therapy can help children replace negative thoughts with more positive interpretations that result in improvements in feelings and behaviors, which in turn has been shown to decrease the risk of depression, anxiety and other problems.

Siblings have their own needs

Inform siblings shortly after the family finds out the diagnosis and be sure to include them in receiving updates over time. Speak with them alone, so they can ask direct questions without trying to protect their brother, to answer their questions and address their concerns. Offer them the opportunity to meet with others outside the family, where they can ask questions not only without worrying about upsetting their brother, but also without worrying about upsetting you. Siblings often feel it is their job to help support their parents and one way to do that may by trying not to burden them with their own concerns. Help them identify ways to get accurate information about their brother's condition and share the same advice on the use of the internet for medical information described earlier.

Be sure to focus some of the conversation on the needs of well siblings for their own personal development. They too have their own needs and aspirations and are deserving of the focused attention of their parents and other family members so they appreciate that they are worthy and important in their own right, not only through the support they provide to their sibling with DMD. Balance offering appropriate ways they can assist their brother with DMD and help their parents with his care, with permission and even encouragement to attend to the well childrens' own personal needs and wants. As older siblings of children with DMD enter adolescence, they may become reluctant to make developmentally appropriate transitions to independence, such as going to college or pursuing a job or career. Be sensitive to this from early on, well before the likely time of transition. There is a big difference between telling children that you really appreciate their watching their brother so you can cook dinner or spend some time with your spouse, and telling children that you don't think you could manage the situation or care for their brother without their help. The latter may make children feel you really can't do it without them and prevent them from pursuing their own education or career out of a profound sense of need and responsibility.

Consider what you will share with peers

It is important to talk with children about what they wish to be shared with teachers, coaches, classmates and others in the community. Having someone talk to the class to share basic information about DMD may minimize teasing by children who don't understand or have no other way to get their questions answered. The focus should be on basic information that is personally relevant to classmates (e.g. that it isn't contagious), as well as the current impact on the child with DMD. With the child's permission, information can be shared about limitations posed by DMD and the current treatments, such as steroids, to the extent that it can explain visible side effects such as weight gain or acne. Children with DMD can be asked whether they would like to be present for the discussion and whether they prefer it to be led by their parent(s), a healthcare professional (such as the school nurse or a member of the team from the medical center), or the teacher (after the teacher has received some background information). These discussions can also help classmates identify ways they can provide effective support to the child with DMD (e.g. offer to help him carry his books; consider ways to engage him in free play that doesn't require as much running; assist him with note taking because of difficulty with maintaining attention in class, etc.). The child with DMD should be asked about what he believes would be helpful. It is important to recognize that at times, parents and other family members may find such public discussion difficult – even when it may be in the best interest of their son, peers and the school staff – because it may require them to confront some of their own distress about their son's illness or their preference for privacy. When this occurs, it is critical to support parents so that they become more comfortable with such sharing, which likely will be relevant to other contexts outside of school, such as professional colleagues at the parent(s)' place of employment and extended family members and friends.

The long-term goal is to increase children's ability to assume an active role in the self-management of their condition and to be in the best position to cope and adjust with the challenges posed over time by the illness and its treatment. Children with DMD are most likely to achieve this goal in the setting of open communication, when surrounded by informed and supportive adults and peers, and when they are shown and able to learn coping techniques.

Chapter Seven

HAVING A ROAD MAP FOR LIFE
Creating an Education, Health and Care Plan for Duchenne Muscular Dystrophy

Nick Catlin

Introduction

Everyone has a life plan. It might be daydreaming about your hopes for the future, a new job or moving house. It could be a few bullet points on a scrap of paper. Today many of us use Google Calendar or other nifty software tools to plan events, mark birthdays or organise complicated work schedules.

What sort of plan do we need with young people living with Duchenne muscular dystrophy? Who should be involved and how can we make sure it gets funded?

For parents, the diagnosis of Duchenne muscular dystrophy is an unexpected shock. It's impossible to forget the day of diagnosis when you are told that your son has a severe muscle wasting condition that is not going to get better. All because of some tiny mutation in a gene that means his muscle cells break down and eventually will not be replaced. He will be in a wheelchair and lose all of his normal muscle function in late teens (Bushby *et al.* 2010a, 2010b; Treat-nmd. eu 2016).

As you have discovered throughout this book, children with DMD are also at risk of neuro-developmental, emotional and behavioural impairments such as autism, ADHD and dyslexia (Ricotti *et al.* 2015). These problems impact on the development of the young person's social, emotional and communication skills. They are also on a spectrum with some young people slightly affected and others with more severe lagging skills.

It all seems so unfair, unreal and at odds with the little boy running around at 3 or 4 years of age, then going to school and having fun with his friends. Caring, teaching and helping that young person through the tough times ahead are the big worries for Mums and Dads. The impact of Duchenne on the family is significant and the levels of support often locked down in multi-agency bureaucracy or lack of funding. However, the good news is that some young people are living longer with Duchenne (Villanova and Kazibwe 2017) and new drugs and treatments are in the pipeline. It is now even more important to think about the longer term and into adulthood.

You need a plan! A road map for life. In some countries, England in the UK for example, there is legislation requiring Education Health and Care Plans (EHC Plans) to be in place. The examples here are from our experience in the UK but the principles apply to wherever you might live.

Wikis, wallpaper and co-production

It is essential to the production of a plan that the young person is able to take a lead and always remain central to the planning process. This ensures that the plan is anchored by the aspirations, dreams and hopes of the young person and focuses on how to help them learn the skills they need to get to where they want to go. The ultimate aim, however, is for the co-production of EHC Plans that include input from the young person, parents, other family members, the community, professional assessments and local authorities.

Agree a good place to meet up. It could be at home or more likely at school or college. Decide who needs to be present at your meeting. Who would the young person like to be there? Who are the stakeholders in supporting and helping this young person to develop their plan? What is your circle of support? Family and community members can offer a great deal towards a plan as well as key education, health and social services professionals.

Begin planning with the young person (Sanderson 2013) and listen. A most important step is for the young person to be prepared to start the meeting. This can be organised as a simple PowerPoint presentation that the young person has developed and can include photos or other media. Some families, particularly in cases where the young person may struggle to convey their thoughts and feelings verbally, choose to use a Wiki instead.

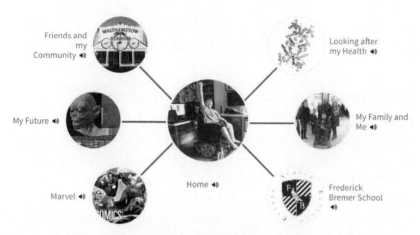

Figure 7.1 Saul's Wiki.
(Reproduced with permission of Saul Catlin)

Wikis have been developed by the Rix Centre at the University of East London in partnership with adults and young people with Special Educational Needs and Disability (Rix Centre UEL 2016). A Wiki is a small website that is secure, owned by the young person and can have multimedia pages that can record the dreams, hopes, aspirations and useful information about the young person living with Duchenne. You can scan or upload PDFs of all those medical, education and social care assessments and have them on your the Wiki. This saves carrying around huge files and losing key documents. It is possible for the young person and their family to give varying levels of access to the Wiki to other members of the family, friends and professionals who might attend the meeting.

This Wiki gives the young person, even those with severe communication problems, the chance to share photos, video clips and web links at the start of a meeting (see 'Sharing Shane's Wiki' on the Rix Centre website (Rix Centre UEL 2016)).

It sets the context for the plan by understanding All About Me and the young person's hopes and dreams for the future. My advice to professionals is to put your files of assessments and learning targets back in your bag and listen. To parents – encourage and help the young person to express himself and try not to squash his ideas or pop his dreams. The Wikis become very personal albums of everyday life and form a real context for developing your plan. But it's OK to start with big sheets of wallpaper and a few marker pens. The most important thing is to encourage empathy with the young person, to listen carefully, acknowledge and record his views.

Structure of the Plan and the Education, Health and Care Plan legislation in England

We recommend that all young people diagnosed with Duchenne Muscular Dystrophy are assessed as soon as possible for an Education Health and Care Plan. In England this requires the young person to have a learning disability or disability that requires SEN provision (see p.91 The final plan and review). The initial referral is usually made by the school SENCO but parents can make a direct request to their Local Authority who must then initiate assessments for a Plan. The initial or review meeting will usually have an agreed structure that can help to guide the development of a written plan. This is essentially a step to informing the writing of the official Education Health and Care (EHC) Plan draft document and is best coordinated by one designated official from the local authority.

The sheets of paper can have headings in areas like the example here from Preparing for Adulthood (2017; see also Preparingforadulthood. org.uk 2016). This format can be used for younger people, even at the early stages of Duchenne.

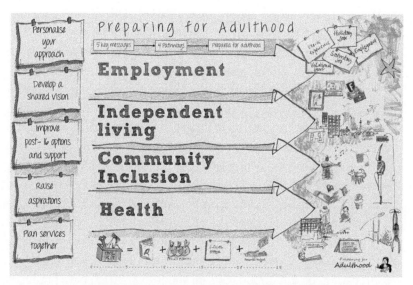

Figure 7.2 Education Health and Care Plan graphics.
(Designed by John Ralphs for Preparing for Adulthood (www. preparingforadulthood.org.uk))

The four key areas in a plan are: Employment/Education, Independent Living, Community Inclusion/Relationships and Health Pathways. Finding out about young people's aspirations in the context of these pathways gives a structure to the plan and helps to advise the final outcomes.

Most 5- or 6-year-olds will tell you what they want to be when they grow up. Obviously this becomes more important to the young person as they grow older and leave formal education, but the Employment/Education pathway at a young age puts into context basic skills that are taught at school including reading, maths, writing, etc. that will be essential for the future.

Independent Living is a key pathway to explore with young people living with Duchenne. It might involve the use of their wheelchair, adaptations to home, access to transport and so on.

Community Inclusion/Relationships is about friends, engaging in local activities, getting out and about, joining clubs and hobbies. Local authorities in England now have to have a Local Offer that gives information about local education, health and social care provision. Check this out by going to your local authority's website and looking at the Local Offer link.

Finally, the Health Pathway needs to explore the best practice for managing Duchenne (Treat-nmd.eu 2016). This needs to include assessments and reports from neuromuscular centres, clinicians, physiotherapists, occupational therapists, respiratory consultants, cardiologists, endocrinologists, nutritionists, psychologists, your GP and any other professionals or agencies involved in supporting the health of the young person. It needs to include information on current medicines that the young person is taking, risk assessments and reference to the Duchenne A and E pack and Emergency App (AandE App Duchenne Muscular Dystrophy 2015). You *must* always discuss medication with your doctor or clinician before taking any drugs, supplements or undertaking interventions.

We have now explored the aspirations of the young person and heard from family, community members and professionals. The planning has been shaped by reference to four key life pathways.

Preparing for Adulthood (Gitsam and Jordan 2015) have produced an excellent summary of person-centred thinking tools and how to use them for EHC planning. There is a comprehensive guide in the toolkit on how to complete the official form for Sections A–K by using person-centred planning methods (Gitsam and Jordan 2015, p.17). IPSEA have also produced a very helpful checklist that families can use to make sure that you have everything covered (IPSEA 2014).

Stay Solution Focused

It's easy to get bogged down with problems. In the worst cases this can end up with blame all round for what is going wrong and the plan comes to a halt and bridges are burned.

Best hopes

When we have been working with families and schools we have taken a Solution Focused approach. Leaning on the philosophy and practice of the Brief Team (Brief.org.uk 2016) and Steve de Shazer (de Shazer and Berg 1997) we have always listened carefully to concerns and gripes but have tried to steer discussion by considering families' and professionals' best hopes.

Try starting your planning session or review with the question:

> *'What are your best hopes for us working together on this plan?'*

or:

> *'What are your best hopes for the outcomes of this review meeting?'*

'Best hopes' questions immediately focus attention on aspirations rather than problems.

Mum: He's always stuck in the house (problem) but I hope that we can all find some ways to get him out more

SENCO: If you were not at home all day Jimmy what would you be doing?

Jimmy: Dunno. Maybe go to the cinema.

Now Jimmy has the opportunity to think about the first steps that he needs to take to get to the cinema. What's on? What are your favourite films? Could he take a friend? How will he handle the money? Can he take the bus? Can he do this without his Mum? What does Jimmy think are the first small steps?

Scaling

Black and white thinkers and those that tend to be inflexible often use catastrophic language or express themselves in very rigid terms when dealing with problems. 'I'll never do that' 'It was so bad I thought I would die', etc. Scaling helps to look for solutions as there are usually some steps that have been achieved, however small. These provide a starting point for moving forward.

Dad: My best hope for Billy is that he learns to read so that he can use the internet and read books for pleasure.

Billy: I'm rubbish and can't read anything. I hate reading. I feel sick when I read.

Special Educational Needs Coordinator (SENCO): If 10 was reading books like Harry Potter and zero was not being able to read anything at all, where would you be on this scale? (You can draw this scale.)

Billy: I'm rubbish so a three.

SENCO: A three? So what can you do right now that makes it a three?

Billy: Well…I can sound out some letters and I can read signs on shops sometimes.

SENCO: That's great. So what do you think you need to do to make it a 4?

Billy: Dunno really. Learn more sounds and then figure out the words.

SENCO: Great. We can get started right away if you like as I have a brilliant programme to help you do just that.

Focusing on aspirations and solutions helps to find out what small steps the young person, perhaps with support, needs to take to get to where he wants to go. Just identifying problems can lead to loss of self esteem, demoralisation and blaming people for what's not working. Solution Focused approaches also lead more readily to identifying SMART (Specific, Measurable, Assignable, Realistic and Time Framed) outcomes.

Assessments to be included in my Plan

Duchenne muscular dystrophy is a complex medical condition and requires carefully considered assessment and follow-up interventions to manage physical and mental health issues undertaken at specialist Centres of Excellence. The muscle wasting is progressive and health management changes over time and will impact on walking, breathing and the heart. New treatments and better management are already changing the course of the condition and so any plan will need to consider and reflect the changing treatment regimes. New genetic treatments, for example, are in the pipeline with Translarna being the first novel drug approved in the UK for funding by NICE in 2016.

Assessments from specialist neuromuscular centres and other consultants will need to be carefully considered by the SENCO and family and how interventions such as physiotherapy, for example, are put in place at a local level. These assessments should be summarised and included as Health Outcomes in the plan. The Duchenne Family Guide is an important place to start. (Treat-nmd.eu 2016)

However, it is not only health assessments that will be necessary for the EHC Plan. In order to think about the four outcomes a range of assessments may well be necessary, depending on the needs of the young person.

As you have read so far, Duchenne muscular dystrophy is also recognised as a neuro-developmental impairment with higher risk of attention deficit/hyperacvitity disorder (ADHD), autism, obsessive-compulsive disorder (OCD) and reading difficulties as well as possible adjustment difficulties (Ricotti *et al.* 2015).

Who to refer to for assessment and diagnosis for these conditions can depend on the area (and country) you live in. In the UK, assessments for learning and cognition are usually carried out by an educational psychologist, and those for behavioural or mental health-related difficulties by a clinical psychologist in a local Child and Adolescent Mental Health Services (CAMHS) team. Referrals can be made by school or your local GP. In the U.S. an assessment by a neuro-psychologist is recommended as this professional will have a better understanding of the impact of neurological differences on learning and behaviour.

These are some of the specific assessments that need to be considered. However, there may be others and so it is always important to talk to your neuromuscular consultant at the muscle clinic or SENCO at school with regard to any issues you are worried about; they should be able to refer you to the relevant service for assessment.

1. Speech and/or language delay or disorder

Boys with DMD are at risk of speech and language delay and so an early assessment by a speech therapist and early intervention are essential if there are concerns (Cyrulnik *et al.* 2007). Often a speech therapist will train a teaching assistant at school on how to implement a programme or lead a group. Your plan needs to mention that any programme needs to be designed by a qualified speech and language therapist and regularly assessed and monitored by them.

2. Assessments for ADHD, ADD, ASD, OCD and working memory

As has been discussed in detail in Chapter 5, some boys with Duchenne can be easily distracted, prone to emotional 'meltdowns', or find it difficult to complete or stay on tasks and can appear stubborn and inflexible. James Poysky says that it is important to see this as 'a cognitive weakness rather than a character flaw' (Poysky 2011, p.22) and to identify how to support a young person to develop these skills.

Ross Greene describes these problems as lagging skills and has developed a useful checklist called the Assessment of Lagging Skills and Underlying Problems (ALSUP) that can be used as a starting point for discussion (Greene 2017).

Problems with working memory have been shown to be a high risk in DMD (Hinton *et al.* 2000, 2001 and 2007; Ricotti *et al.* 2015). Working memory is a concept that describes how we process information on a temporary basis and relay it to and fro into long-term memory storage for a whole range of cognitive tasks (Baddeley 1992). These can be tasks such as managing phonics and basic number skills. It can include managing conversations and processing lists of instructions. Young people that have these working memory problems need well designed and systematic interventions with lots of deliberate practice (Ericsson and Pool 2017) to make sure that they develop the cognitive skills they need for reading writing, and numbers.

Susan Gathercole and Tracy Packiam Alloway have developed a basic guide with good general tips about understanding and supporting children with working memory problems (Gathercole and Packiam Alloway 2007). There are paper and pencil tests available in the Working Memory Test Battery for Children, which is standardised for children aged 4 to 15 years. They have also developed a simple PC-based program called the Automated Working Memory Assessment (AWMA) that can be used from 4 to 22 years (Gathercole and Packiam Alloway 2007, p.11).

3. Social communication and making friends

As well as physical challenges making it difficult for boys to be included in peer games, boys with DMD can find it difficult to make and maintain friendships due to social communication difficulties. Boys with DMD are at higher risk of ASD (see Chapters 1 and 4) and OCD. A referral to CAMHS, a clinical psychologist or your Community Mental Health Team for assessment is an important consideration. See Chapter 5 for suggestions on interventions for skills to help to develop friendships.

4. Coping emotionally and adjusting to Duchenne

Some boys have difficulty coping emotionally with their deteriorating condition and may need assessment and intervention from the Community Mental Health Team who might refer them for counselling or coaching.

5. Reading, spelling, writing and numbers

Some boys with Duchenne have problems learning to read and spell. They can have problems writing longer sentences and constructing essay-type answers to questions. These boys might also have difficulties with maths and processing numbers.

It is important to look specifically at assessments for phonics, single word reading, spelling and number skills. Assessments for learning that just report on overall IQ scores are of little value. We need more fine-tuned evaluations that are going to pinpoint both strengths and lagging skills. From this point appropriate interventions can be designed and implemented.

Research has suggested that carefully constructed interventions, with lots of short but intensive repetition, can make a considerable difference (Hoskin and Fawcett 2014). See Chapter 4 for a more detailed discussion on interventions for reading and learning.

6. Assessments for Access Arrangements

Access Arrangements are special arrangements that can be put in place for any young person in the UK who needs extra time or support in formal examinations, for example with reading, writing or with the use of a computer. In order to qualify, the young person must have an assessment by a qualified specialist teacher or psychologist and achieve below a certain level in recognised tests (Jcq.org.uk 2017). Using a scribe in lessons and for exams is a very useful way to ensure that the young person with Duchenne is getting down on paper their knowledge and understanding of a subject. Providing writing frames or a list of key sentences helps to get the young person started on longer writing tasks.

Results of any formal assessments for the above (and any more) must be included in Section B of the EHC Plan relating to a young person's Special Educational Needs and Disability .

Crucially the EHC Plan must also consider outcomes in all these areas that will help the young person to practise and improve their lagging skills whether they are in communication, reading, learning or concentration.

Outcomes

What is an outcome and what is the process for defining them for young people with Duchenne? In the SEND Code outcomes are key and are the basis on which provision is made and resources allocated.

Outcomes must be SMART. In other words they should be specific, measurable, assignable, realistic and time related. Don't accept woolly outcomes or vague statements. You need to know what the young person is going to do and with whom in an agreed time frame. You need to work out how success will be measured. It can be helpful to get started by setting outcomes in a grid like Table 7.1, which is for a younger child with DMD.

Table 7.1 Sample outcomes grid for a younger child with DMD

My Future	What small steps will you achieve now and in the next 3–12 months	Who will do it with you?	By when?	What resources will you need?	How will we know if it's successful?	How well did we succeed?
Education Learning and Employment	For Brian to be able to recognise and sound out all the 44 phonemes.	Class teacher, TA, parents and grandparents.	Feb. 2016	Read Write Inc. scheme, or synthetic reading scheme, flash cards, books.	Brian can recognise and sound out all 44 phonemes for reading.	Brian can now recognise 23 phonemes with regular success. See assessment sheet.
Friends, Relationships and Community	Brian to meet on a weekly basis with a small group of peers who are good and confident communicators with an adult facilitator so that he can make more friends and be better able to manage everyday conversations.	Facilitator, class teacher, TA, circle of friends.	Feb. 2016	Facilitator training and setting up the group. Room booking.	Brian has become more self-confident and has a wider group of friends that he is able to play with and make conversations on a number of topics. Has fewer aggressive outbursts with classmates.	Brian has made one good friend from the group but still finds it hard to make conversation and still has regular meltdowns over small issues.
Living Independently	Family to make suitable adaptations to home so that Brian has access to his own wet room, toilet and the garden.	Parents, local authority grant application, OT.	Nov. 2016	Completed grant application for building works.	Brian has full access to downstairs in the house with use of a wet room and toilet. He can also safely use the garden.	The application for a grant has has been submitted but funding has yet to be agreed.
Health	To attend a 6-monthly review at Great Ormond Street Hospital Neuromuscular service.	Parents, Neuromuscular Team	23rd March 2016	Transport to GOSH and arrange an overnight stay in London.	Physiotherapy North Star Assessment completed. Review of steroid medication. Breathing assessment. Prophylactic heart medication reviewed.	Physiotherapy advice from GOSH and physical management programme has not been implemented by local service. Heart medication increased dose. Sleep study recommended.

You can have *more than one outcome* for the four areas but try to keep to the key objectives of your plan. The Council for Disabled Children (2017), Preparing for Adulthood (2017) and the UK Department for Education (Department for Education and Department of Health 2014) provide some good resources and examples of best practice for identifying Outcomes in their Code of Practice.

Risk assessments

Think about having risk assessments as part of your plan. Most local authorities, schools and colleges have risk assessments in place and templates and policies (e.g. Risk Assessments Hertfordshire Grid 2016) that can be adapted. The Health and Safety Executive has information for manual handling (Manual Handling HSE 2016).

The risk assessments that need to be included in the plan are those specifically related to the young person with Duchenne. The best risk assessments are those co-produced between staff at school or college, the young person and their family, and professionals like OTs and physiotherapists. They should identify levels of risk and how these risks will be managed.

The most common risks to be considered are falling or injuries in the playground or when using play equipment for younger boys. It does not mean boys with Duchenne should be excluded from PE or physical activity but rather wherever possible the risks involved, how they will be managed and who is involved should be identified. Trips out or residentials need specific risk assessments. Into adulthood, risks involving manual handling, hoisting, transfers and transport for example need to be considered.

Safeguarding issues are important for young people with DMD particularly as they get older and need help with personal care (Murray 2009). It is important they are supported to say no if and when they are not happy with the support they are receiving.

Mitigating risks might require writing specific outcomes for a plan and these might need resources and funding further in the plan. For example, one or more TAs might be employed at lunchtimes to supervise playground and play equipment activities used by a boy with Duchenne. It will be important to carefully define the person's role and how the risks will be managed. Staff, the young person, the family and if need be outside professionals should be involved in co-production. It is not possible to identify all risks, and remember risk assessments should written to ensure young disabled people are as independent as possible and that they have the right to be involved and enjoy as many as possible of the activities and events that are open to their non-disabled peers.

The final Plan and reviews (for England only)

Final Plans can become statutory documents that require local authorities by law to provide specialist provision and interventions. In England, for example, the legislation for Education Health and Care Plans require local authorities to complete a template with sections ranging from A to K. The template may vary and might not be in use for your child's school or college but the template from the Code of Practice does serve as a good example of how a Plan might be formally structured. Table 7.2 includes some comments and ideas that can help guide families and young people living with Duchenne. For a full checklist with notes on relevant sections from the Code please refer to the excellent IPSEA Guide (IPSEA 2014)

Table 7.2 Checklist for EHC Plan

		Duchenne Muscular Dystrophy Notes
SECTION A	The views, interests and aspirations of the child or young person and their parents.	This is your chance to record your aspirations, hopes and dreams for the future. It can be a summary of your Wiki and your Person Centred Planning meeting. It usually has a one-page summary.
SECTION B	The child or young person's Special Educational Needs.	A Special Educational Need is a learning difficulty or disability that needs SEN provision. Think of it as a list of impairments that are a result of living with Duchenne muscular dystrophy. These will be identified through assessments by education and health professionals. SEN may include needs for health and social care provision that are treated as special educational provision because they educate or train a child or young person (see paragraphs 9.73 of the SEN Code onwards. https://www.gov.uk/government/publications/send-code-of-practice-0-to-25). The SEN provision, in the case of Duchenne, can involve extra support to manage the risks of falling, for trips and visits, personal care, to access the school curriculum and exams, to undertake specialist programmes, etc. It can involve direct intervention from specialists such as physiotherapists, OTs, speech therapists and literacy and numeracy teachers.
SECTION C	The child or young person's health care needs which relate to their SEN.	Use the family guide (Duchenne Family Guide 2016)) to check that you have included all aspects of management of the young person's medical condition. Refer to reports from neuromuscular consultants, physiotherapists, cardiologists, respiratory consultants, endocrinologists etc to summarise the young persons Health Needs. Include medication and Accident and Emergency advice (AandE App Duchenne Muscular Dystrophy 2015). Include any reports or assessments by Clinical or Educational Psychologists for neuro-developmental disorders such as ADHD, ASD and for depression. You must always discuss medication with your doctor or clinician before taking any drugs, supplements or undertaking interventions.
SECTION D	The child or young person's social care needs which relate to their SEN or to a disability.	An EHC Plan in England must include a statutory assessment of the young person's social care needs. A social worker will be designated (or more likely you have to contact social services yourself) to assess the young person's needs and this will trigger a discussion about personal assistant (PA) support, short breaks provision and funding. Any outcomes from risk assessments.

SECTION E	The outcomes sought for the child or young person (including outcomes for life).	Make sure that you get this right. These are the longer-term outcomes or goals and must be SMART and reflect everything that has been written in Section A. Create outcomes within the four strands of: 1. Employment, Education and Training 2. Health 3. Independent Living 4. Friendships, Relationships and Community Inclusion. Any outcomes from risk assessments.
SECTION F	The special educational provision required by the child or young person	Provision or interventions are linked to longer-term outcomes. In fact they should be written as short term SMART outcomes: 1. Employment, Education and Training 2. Health 3. Independent Living 4. Friendships, Relationships and Community Inclusion. They have to be specific and support the young person to gain new skills in order to achieve their goals in life. Specify who is going to make this provision and for how many hours per week. Work out the costs. Therapies such as physiotherapy, or CAHMS (Child and Adult Mental Health Services) must appear in this section as well as in health care. 'Once specified in this section, the LA must "secure" the provision, i.e. they must ensure that it is made. If a health body ceases to make the provision, the duty falls on the [local authority] LA. An LA may well delegate funding to a school or post 16 institution, but if those institutions cannot make the provision out of that funding, then the LA is legally obliged to do so (s.42 Children and Families Act 2014)' (IPSEA 2014). Any outcomes from risk assessments.
SECTION G	Any health provision reasonably required by the learning difficulties or disabilities which result in the child or young person having SEN	Health provision must be detailed and specific. It should be clear how the provision is meeting the best practice medical care for Duchenne, who is providing it and for how long. Where possible work out the costs involved. The young person might require a Continuing Health Care Assessment (CHC) (Nhs.uk 2016) that assesses those with severe health needs. Any outcomes from risk assessments.

cont.

	Duchenne Muscular Dystrophy Notes	
SECTION H1	Any social care provision which must be made for a child or young person under 18 resulting from s.2 Chronically Sick and Disabled Persons Act (CSDPA) 1970.	Section H1 of the EHC Plan must specify all services assessed as being needed for a disabled child or young person under 18, under section 2 of the Chronically Sick and Disabled Persons Act (CSDPA)1970. These services include: • practical assistance in the home • provision or assistance in obtaining recreational and educational facilities at home and outside the home • assistance in travelling to facilities • adaptations to the home • facilitating the taking of holidays • provision of meals at home or elsewhere • provision or assistance in obtaining a telephone and any special equipment necessary • non-residential short breaks (included in Section H1 on the basis that the child as well as his or her parent will benefit from the short break). Work out the costs involved. Any outcomes from risk assessments.
SECTION H2	Any other social care provision reasonably required by the learning difficulties or disabilities which result in the child/young person having SEN.	'Social care provision contained in Section H2 will be any other social care provision reasonably required (by the child or young person's learning difficulties or disabilities which result in SEN). Note that this is only provision "reasonably" required, so LAs can take into account cost and convenience, unlike the provision in Section F. If the child is in or beyond Year 9 (broadly speaking, 14 years old or older) the social care provision required to assist in the preparation for adulthood and independent living must be included here. For example, support in finding employment, housing or for participation in society' (IPSEA 2014). Any outcomes from risk assessments.
SECTION I	Placement	The name and type of the school, maintained nursery school, post 16 institution or other institution to be attended by the child or young person.
SECTION J	Personal budget (including arrangements for direct payments).	This is where the individual budget is specified. Make sure that the budget or costs are linked to short-term SMART Outcomes identified in Section F. Ask for a breakdown of costs relating to a personal budget. How will these payments be monitored and paid?
SECTION K	Advice and information	Attach copies of reports, assessments, advice and information.

The budget – linking provision to costs

The key step in developing your plan is to make sure that the interventions or provisions are linked to the outcomes and they must be costed. In the tables below are some examples (*not* a full plan) from Simon's EHC Plan. Simon, aged 16 years, has Duchenne muscular dystrophy and wants to attend his local Sixth Form College to study while living with his family at home.

Budgets for SEND provision are developed by local authorities and are held by schools and colleges in England. This has been agreed so that schools and colleges can provide and train support staff and specialist teachers. It is important in your plan to break down the interventions or provision and ensure that it is costed and going to be made by the school or college. Co-production with the local authority and school or college staff, usually the SENCO, is essential to make sure resources are in place.

Section F Educational Provisions linked to Outcomes – Table 7.3 includes some examples for transition to FE or Sixth Form at 16 years from secondary school for a young person living with Duchenne. These examples can be adapted for younger people or adults depending on need.

Table 7.3 Exemplar Section F for EHC plan for a 16-year-old with DMD

Education Intervention (linked to Outcome)	Who will provide this?	Cost
A college environment which is wheelchair friendly and has access to all classrooms and college facilities.	Sixth Form College	College organisation – reasonable adjustments.
PA support to enable me to use public transport to get to and from college daily, consistent with the 'assistance with travel policy'.	To be determined by family from their personal budget	A budget can be allocated to family instead of using local authority special transport arrangements (specify £)*.
PA support to enable me to join in college trips and to access local activities during college time.	Sixth Form College	College organisation – reasonable adjustments or allocated budget (specify £)*.

cont.

Education Intervention (linked to Outcome)	Who will provide this?	Cost
PA support at college with my personal care as needed to include toileting.	Sixth Form College	To be determined out of funding (specify £)* allocated to college for personal care.
Support to take up work experience and internship during term time.	Sixth Form College	To be covered by college using the element 2 funding within the budget (specify £)*.
LSA or TA in-class support for all my 13 timetabled sessions for the IT course to ensure that I understand instructions, scribe and complete assignment. Where possible, I should access my curriculum in standing position.	Sixth Form College	To be covered by college using the element 3 funding (specify £)*.
A teacher or LSA support one to one for 3 hours per week outside of classes to help me organise my projects and assignments, understand examination criteria and scribe especially when I am required to write lots of information. This should include support for my main IT course, with English skills development incorporated in this.	Sixth Form College	To be covered by college using the element 3 funding (specify £)*.
Access support for exams is essential. My requirements are as follows: 50 per cent extra time, a scribe, a reader to explain complex information, and a computer.	Sixth Form College	College organisation – reasonable adjustments.
Individual adult support and supervision to transfer into standing position using my sit-to-stand wheelchair, up to 60 minutes a day depending on my tolerance, as part of my 24 hour postural management programme. Where possible I should access my curriculum in standing position.	Sixth Form College	College – to be covered using element 2 and 3 funding (specify £)*
To complete a risk assessment for College that will include at least: manual handling, emergency evacuation, A and E Emergency admissions to hospital, trips outside of College.	Sixth Form College	College organisation – reasonable adjustments.

*It is important to specify exactly the amount of funding that is being used to deliver support or interventions for the young person. This is often granted from the local authority in a funding allocation to meet all Special Educational Needs in a school or college. Ask exactly how much of this funding is being allocated to meet the needs of the individual young person with Duchenne.

In the UK, the health budgets are commissioned by the National Health Service. There are tertiary specialist services like Neuromuscular Centres of Excellence, secondary hospital services and primary services like GPs and dentists. Each service has its own budgets and commissioners. Costs for specialist neuromuscular services are not usually broken down for EHC Plans but it is essential to include their assessments and agreed interventions in the plan as these need to be reviewed and expert advice followed by local providers. It is the same for secondary and primary NHS services. For Duchenne, the real problem is accessing local physiotherapy services and hydrotherapy. Where possible ask for budgets to ensure this provision is being made and in line with expert advice.

Section G Health Provisions linked to Outcomes – Table 7.4 includes some examples for a young person, aged 16 years, living with Duchenne, but these can be adapted for younger children depending on assessment and age.

You *must* always discuss medication with your doctor or clinician before taking any drugs, supplements or undertaking interventions. It is important to refer to the standards of medical care for Duchenne that have been internationally published and reviewed. These will be periodically updated following research (Treat-nmd.eu 2016; Vry *et al.* 2016).

Table 7.4 Exemplar Section G of EHC plan – some examples for a 16-year-old living with DMD

Health Intervention (linked to Outcome)	Who will provide this?	Cost
I will be supported to attend all medical appointments including 6-monthly reviews at expert Neuromuscular Centre (used GOSH here as an example).	Great Ormond Street Hospital Neuromuscular Team, Parents	Family – any cost to be determined until Continuing Health Care threshold is met by Health

cont.

Health Intervention (linked to Outcome)	Who will provide this?	Cost
I will continue to take my medication as prescribed by my consultants.	Great Ormond Street Hospital Neuromuscular Team, Parents	Cost to be determined by GP and tertiary health services. Family support for medication.
My respirator will be reviewed by the Sleep Unit at Great Ormond Street Hospital.	Great Ormond Street Hospital Neuromuscular Team, Sleep Study Team and Parents	Cost to be determined by Tertiary NHS Service*. Family to support.
I will have continued support with my sleep ventilation programme to help with my breathing at night at home every day.	Parents	Cost to be determined by Tertiary NHS Service. Family to support.
My testosterone injections will be administered, as prescribed every month at the GP clinic.	Great Ormond Street Hospital Neuromuscular Team, Endocrinology Team GOSH, GP, parents	Cost to be determined by Tertiary NHS Service. Family to support.
Zonodronic acid and infusions will be administered and reviewed to minimise bone damage.	Great Ormond Street Hospital Neuromuscular Team, Endocrinology Team GOSH Whipps Cross Hospital, parents	Cost to be determined by Tertiary NHS Service and local NHS Health Budget*. Family to support.
My heart medication will be kept at the optimum level.	Great Ormond Street Hospital Neuromuscular Team, Cardiology Team GOSH, parents	Cost to be determined by Tertiary NHS Service. Family to support.
My diet and exercise will be regularly monitored.	Great Ormond Street Hospital Neuromuscular Team, parents	Cost to be determined by Tertiary NHS Service. Family to support.
Hydrotherapy session once a week for 3 hours (the 3 hours to include lifeguard, travel time, changing time before and after hydrotherapy) and access to a hydrotherapy pool.	PA to support young person (Personal Budget) and hydrotherapy centre	To be funded out of the (specify £)* Short Breaks funding. To be funded out of the (specify £)* per annum paid directly to the Hydrotherapy Centre term time only.

Access to a Paediatric Physiotherapist and 6-monthly reviews to: Monitor and manage my physical condition. Devise the physical management programme. Teach the programme to relevant staff members. Liaise with tertiary/specialist centres and education staff.	Physiotherapy Team	Local Health Budget (specify £)*.

*It is currently difficult to get specific costs allocated to individuals from the UK NHS system as it aims to provide universal health care. It is important to make sure that a young person living with Duchenne attends a Neuromuscular Centre of Excellence and that recommendations are passed to GPs and local services like physiotherapy. Short breaks funding can be used for supporting activities like hydrotherapy and these budgets can be allocated to individuals.

In the UK, young people living with Duchenne are entitled to a social worker. There are also short breaks budgets and domiciliary care budgets available to pay for Personal Assistants (PAs) and carers.

Section H Social Care Provisions linked to Outcomes – Table 6.5 includes some examples from a young person aged 16 years living with Duchenne. These examples can be adapted for younger children and adults.

Table 7.5 Exemplar Section H of EHC Plan – some examples for a 16-year-old living with DMD

Social Care Intervention (linked to Outcome)	Who will provide this?	Cost
To be able to get up in the morning at a time of my choosing, to use the toilet, get dressed, have a shower, have breakfast and be ready for the day's activities. PA support one hour daily (seven days).	PA funded by social services domiciliary care budget.	To be funded out of budget (specify £) for domiciliary care

cont.

Social Care Intervention (linked to Outcome)	Who will provide this?	Cost
To be able to go to bed in the evening at a time of my choosing, use the toilet, get undressed, have a shower and check my respirator PA support one hour daily (seven days).	PA funded by social services domiciliary care budget	To be funded out of (specify £) for domiciliary care.
To have my needs met during the night including relief of cramps and turning in bed and checking my respirator.	Parents	Family – cost to be determined and reviewed.
To be entered on list for specialist housing provisions in the local community by March 2017.	Social worker will liaise with Housing	Social worker costs.
Wheelchairs provided and maintained that meet my daily needs.	Wheelchair services	Local wheelchair services
PA support to enable me to attend activities or events during weekends, college and holiday times to extend my friendship groups and gain new skills.	PA funded by social services short breaks budget	To be covered out of the (specify £) Short Breaks funding.

Personal Budgets

It is now possible to ask for a Personal Budget. Some of the funding for Education, Health and Social Care can be allocated via direct payments to the young person. The advantages are that you can hire your own PAs and buy into interventions or provision that best suit you. Remember that you will become an employer. Disability Rights offers a helpline on Personal Budget issues (Disabilityrightsuk.org 2017).

Summary

- All young people living with Duchenne muscular dystrophy need an Education Health and Care Plan. Start from diagnosis.

- In England there is legislation requiring plans from 0–25 years; however, write one anyway even if there is no legal requirement.

- A plan must be centred on the young person living with Duchenne. Take lots of time to ask young people about their dreams, hopes and aspirations for the future. Listen. Listen. Listen.

- Use a wiki, PowerPoint or sheets of paper to document their responses. What knowledge, information or skills are you going to need find or work on to get to where you want to go? Spotlight their interests, achievements, hobbies, family, circle of friends.

- Get other people to contribute to the plan – they can often be a huge untapped resource. Co-produce your plan with family members, friends from your local community, education, health and social care professionals.

- Identify and agree key Outcomes for Education and Employment; Friends, Relationships and Community Activities; Independent Living; Health.

- Make sure resources, with budgets, are written into your plan so that you have the right support to meet your Outcomes and learn new skills

- Review your plan. You might need to review outcomes in three months or a year. Do more of what is working well and find solutions to any new problems.

Chapter Eight

TAKING CHARGE OF TRANSITION TO ADULTHOOD IN DMD

Janet Hoskin and Celine Barry

Introduction

In this chapter we will be talking about what Transition to Adulthood means, and why it is so important to make this a positive and proactive time in the life of a young person with Duchenne muscular dystrophy (DMD). We will look briefly at the literature relating to Transition and DMD, and what a better medical outlook and the new SEND legislation in England might offer. We will explore the lessons we have learned from managing Action Duchenne's five-year lottery-funded Transition to Adulthood project called 'Takin' Charge', and we will report on what boys and parents think are the most important issues. Finally we will share some case studies of young people and families from the Takin' Charge project, and explore how young people and their families are preparing for the future they want.

What do we mean by Transition to Adulthood?

In the UK, health and social care providers use the term 'Transition' to refer to the time when a disabled young person is 18 years old, and their subsequent transfer from paediatric or children's services to adult health and social care provision. In education, we talk about 'Transition' as the time between Year 9 through to the end of school or Further Education College (aged 14–19 years), where the focus is on 'getting ready' for adulthood. In school, Transition is supposed to enable young people with Special Educational Needs and Disability (SEND) enough time to put into place support and resources to ensure that they can reach outcomes they have identified as important as they become adults, for example, a career they may want to pursue, or a housing option they may want to choose. There have been reservations published about this way of thinking. For example, some have suggested that most young people are often not physically or mentally ready to think about adulthood when they are in their teens, and others have warned that usual teenage routes that place an emphasis on careers and independent living may not be the priorities for young people living with life-limiting impairments (Beresford and Stuttard 2014; Gibson *et al.* 2014).

What does the research tell us about the experience of Transition in DMD?

Published research paints a pretty bleak picture of Transition to Adulthood for adults with DMD in the UK. Between 2007 and 2009, Abbott and Carpenter interviewed 40 adults with DMD and their families about their experience of Transition and found that only one person had gained paid employment, all were living at home with their parents and many had very limited social interaction (Abbott, Carpenter and Bushby 2012). In other literature, adults with DMD are described as marginalised and unanticipated (Rahbek *et al.* 2005; Schrans *et al.* 2013). With the introduction of night ventilation, as well as the use of steroids and heart management young people with DMD are living longer lives (Eagle *et al.* 2007). Average life expectancy is now around 30 years, with some adults living into their forties and even their fifties in some countries. This is not to suggest that DMD is not a life-threatening impairment – it is – and we still see young people in their teens dying from it or its consequences, but with better care and treatments that are now available in many countries the outlook is much brighter.

SEND legislation and Transition

As you have read in earlier chapters, the Children and Families Act (2014) in England highlights the need for us to identify and support better outcomes for young people with SEND. In addition, Chapter 7 of the SEND Code of Practice is now dedicated to Transition and there is a requirement that in preparation for adulthood all young people with SEND discuss their plans for employment, independent living, health and social inclusion (DfE and DoH 2015 7: 38). The possible impact of this for young people with DMD should not be ignored, as there is now an expectation that young people with SEND will be progressing to employment or housing options of their choice. Moreover, due to the Care Act (2014), paediatric health and social care provision must continue until adult provision is in place so there should no longer be the situation where young people and families were literally 'falling off the edge' of the social care system when children and adult services failed to join up (Care Quality Commission 2014).

Furthermore, the new legislation allows for an extension of an Education Health and Care Plan up to the age of 25 years where there is a recognised ongoing need for educational support in preparing for adulthood in order to gain employment or more independence.

Although it's too early to assess long-term impact, recent evaluations indicate a positive response from young people with SEND and families about the new legislation, with evaluations of the Pathfinders Programme showing overall high satisfaction with the changes, and a more recent small scale project reporting that young people and families prefer the new person-centred philosophy (Department for Education 2014, 2015 and 2016).

The Takin' Charge project

The Big Lottery-funded Takin' Charge project that took place between 2011 and 2016 was established therefore in a time of great policy change for disabled young people in England. The aim of this project was to support eighty 14–19-year-olds with DMD to think seriously about their future with regard to careers and housing options, sexual health, medical care and social inclusion. It also supported 80 parents through 'Letting Go' workshops and siblings of boys with DMD through 'What about us' workshops. Key to the development and success of the whole programme was the steering committee – four adults with DMD who helped to support and direct the project.

The project involved boys completing a series of online challenges on an e-portfolio. It was delivered through workshops at Action Duchenne's international conferences and national meetings as well as in partnership with seven children and young people's hospices across the country. We were fortunate to find professionals in a variety of roles who were experienced in supporting disabled young people to get the lives they wanted, including organisations that supported employment, housing, sexual health and advocacy, advice and information.

In addition, boys took part in a range of creative projects. For example, in 2013 they co-produced an animation called 'Living with Duchenne' which gave advice to younger children on how to have the best life possible if you have a life-limiting impairment. This was storyboarded and narrated by the boys themselves in partnership with animation graduates from Central St Martins Arts College, London. The animation can be viewed on the Decipha CIC Youtube channel (Decipha CIC 2014). They worked with a music professional to compose and record the music and lyrics for 'Protest Beats' which were used were used in Action Duchenne's lobbies at Westminster and in the Scottish, Welsh and Northern Irish Parliaments. Some of the boys took part in performance poetry workshops, others explored drama as a way of thinking about future careers. A variety of innovative IT sessions allowed boys to create movie trailers or election manifestos, focusing both on the advocacy skills and support that are necessary to have the best life possible. All of these creative projects were essentially a vehicle to support young people to think seriously about their future.

Letting go for parents

Another aspect of the Takin' Charge project was supporting individual families to navigate the new SEND legislation and the current Equality law. In addition to general signposting workshops, we offered individual person-centred planning sessions for those families whose young people were about to leave school. Usually these took part at home as a 'dry-run' for the meetings at school, but sometimes we attended the statutory meetings to offer support.

When we started the project in 2011, our focus was very much solely on the boys. We saw 'independence' as boys thinking about their futures and making plans away from their parents, and we organised workshops so that parents and young people were separated. However, it soon became clear to us that the boys who were able to achieve their identified outcomes most successfully, were those whose parents had been present or very actively involved in supporting them, and so we began to combine many of the sessions. Sexual Health workshops were always for young people only, and sessions on Coping as a Parent were delivered exclusively for parents.

The steering committee

Our steering committee of adults living with DMD consisted regularly of four adults aged between 21 and 45 years old, but sometimes additional volunteers would join for a one-off meeting. The committee helped to develop the direction of the project as well as plan events, and was crucial in working with speakers from other voluntary organisations. The success of the steering committee is illustrated in the setting up of a new charity called DMD Pathfinders which is the first charity run by people with DMD for people with DMD. The importance of this organisation should not be underestimated – until now what has constituted 'user led' has been organisations with parent board members, or more recently, organisations which have been set up and managed by parents themselves. Incredible work has been achieved and continues to be done by these people, but now for the first time we are hearing the voice of people who are actually living with the impairment which cannot be ignored.

Sex and sexuality

If young people with DMD aspire to a full adult life then this should include opportunities to explore sex, sexuality and relationships. The Family Planning Association (FPA) who have experience of delivering sex education to young people and parents across the UK, worked with our steering committee to develop an appropriate and relevant sex and sexuality programme for DMD.

We had not anticipated that members of the steering committee themselves would want some support in this area. Consequently, separate sessions were designed and delivered for older members of Takin' Charge and the steering committee in collaboration with the

FPA and later with the College of Sex and Relationship Therapists (COSRT). These included input from both sex therapists and volunteer adults with DMD. The sessions provided the opportunity for adults with DMD to explore and receive relevant information about relationships, intimacy and sexuality. Evaluations indicate that these workshops were very well received, and offered something that had never been addressed for these young adults.

At the same time as we were progressing this work, the Takin' Charge team became involved with a multi-disciplinary group led by the Open University in the UK (a public distance learning and research university) in partnership with Together for Short Lives (the leading Children's Hospice Movement). These organisations formed a Sexuality Alliance in recognition of the need for sexuality resources for professionals supporting young people with life-limiting conditions (LLCs). Through involvement in this Alliance, Takin' Charge contributed to the production and dissemination of Guidance and Standards for those talking about sex, sexuality and relationships with young people with life-limiting conditions (Open University 2016). There is still much to be done in this area and we are pleased that DMD Pathfinders are progressing this work.

The use of solution focused approaches

Solution Focused Brief Therapy (SFBT) is a form of therapy developed by Steve de Shazer in Milwaukee in the 1980s and which is now quite widely used in the UK. The idea of SFBT is to focus on constructing solutions rather than resolving problems. It assumes that people want to find solutions and are in fact already involved in successful ways of working. In the project we did not offer therapy, but we did employ solution focused approaches wherever possible. This isn't to say we attempted to trivialise the challenges people were facing, nor were we suggesting that people just needed to sort themselves out and stop complaining.

As others have argued, resilience isn't something we are born with, but is affected by the support and resources that are at our disposal, be they material or emotional. This is particularly true now when austerity narratives seek to depict disabled people and their families as to blame for difficult situations they may find themselves in

(Runswick-Cole and Goodley 2013). We started from the viewpoint that parents and young people are the experts of their own lives and are often achieving what works well for them to some degree. We also encouraged young people and families to think about what they wanted to see in their lives in the future, and how what they were doing in the present was helping to achieve this. In other words, identifying what is working well and doing more of it. Most powerfully of all, we encouraged young people and their parents to think about when they would be 25 years old and what they hoped they would be doing.

We were also fully aware of Georgina Eakes' ideas about Chronic Sorrow which suggest that for families affected by life-limiting impairments, grief can be cyclical and can raise its head at times when we are forced to face the full implications of diagnosis, such as at hospital appointments or when our children reach a particular milestone like becoming a teenager or losing the ability to walk (Eakes, Burke and Hainsworth 1998). So we wanted to support families to realise how strong they were at dealing with these difficult issues in their lives while at the same time offering support and information that would equip them for getting the help their young people needed. An important part of most of our workshops therefore was offering parents the chance to share parenting and support skills, as well possible routes to gaining resources and navigating services.

Not forgetting siblings

It can be difficult and frustrating for siblings of young people with DMD who may feel as though their needs are overlooked. Hospital and school appointments can sometimes seem endless and siblings can often be either dragged along or left with a neighbour or family member. Older siblings can sometimes feel embarrassed about having a brother who is 'different' and then feel guilty for their embarrassment. Through the Takin' Charge project we benefited from the input of a national organisation for siblings of disabled children, called 'Sibs', who were able to explore with parents the issues involved in meeting the needs of their other children. We also offered workshops for siblings at national conferences and meetings that were delivered by trained sibling support workers. These workshops involved activities that allowed siblings to think about their own emotional well-being through fun activities that involved discussing feelings. Workshop leaders were also able to share important information about DMD in a safe and creative way.

In one of the hospices that we partnered, a group of older siblings in their twenties were keen to find out about genetic counselling and the possibility of their being carriers of DMD. Due to this need we engaged the services of a genetic counsellor who ran sessions for DMD carriers in our conferences and helped us to co-create a leaflet about being a carrier (Kenwrick 2016).

Feedback from evaluations of Takin' Charge

We conducted interviews and focus groups with parents, steering committee members and the boys who took part in the project. The findings from the parent interviews have recently been published and it is hoped that the boys and adults' views will be published in the future (Hoskin 2017).

The importance of older role models

Both boys and parents reported that key to the success of the project was the involvement of older men with DMD who were able to share their journey to adulthood. For some adults this had meant going to university and starting work, for others it had meant achieving a care package and a flat so that they could live independently, for others it had meant becoming more confident to ask for the support they needed. Parents in particular said that being able to get to know adults with DMD, who may have been using full time ventilation or PEG bags or a variety of technological supports, which in the past they would have found frightening, challenged their ideas and expectations for the future. Before hearing from these adults, parents said that they may well have assumed that achieving employment or independent living would be impossible. But hearing their stories made them realise that often these interventions did not define them, and in fact often supported them to achieve their dreams.

Meeting other families

Parents also reported that meeting other families had been incredibly important to them, and many viewed other parents as the real specialists in DMD who could share ideas about obtaining resources. Boys reported the importance of meeting friends, particularly as being a wheelchair user can exclude you from accessing non-disabled friends' houses or meeting venues.

Getting the resources for a 'normal life'

Parents and boys also reported on their need to get a 'normal life' that could involve the sort of things other non-disabled teenagers might aspire to such as employment, friendship groups and housing and doing what they considered to be 'normal things'. Both boys and parents talked about the importance of having a plan, particularly when living with a complex impairment which often included the involvement of many services and a range of professionals. Some parents felt that they wanted to re-establish their parent relationship rather than simply being carers so benefited from the signposting workshops from various support agencies that were on offer.

The importance of high expectations and planning

The adults with DMD who were part of the steering committee discussed how different the prognosis is now for young people with DMD, and how they might have planned their lives differently had they known they had so many more years to live than anyone had anticipated. For them, their lives had very much been about living from day to day without any major life plans, and yet despite this at least one of them had gone on to university and gained employment. However, he acknowledged how different the journey could have been if he had a plan, and how many more young people with DMD may well have done the same as him if they had been better supported to do so.

All of this seems to contrast with findings from adults with DMD in Canada (Gibson *et al.* 2014). In interviews with 10 adults with DMD, Gibson and colleagues recommend that perhaps the usual trajectory of college to employment and residential independence may not be the most suitable route for those with a life-limiting impairment like DMD. Gibson quotes an adult they interviewed in 2007 talking about 'making the most of the time I have left' rather than focusing on issues such as finding a job or a place to live. Whereas our evaluations of Takin' Charge suggested that young people with DMD and their parents saw their career aspirations or ideas about independent living as an important part of 'making the most of life'. They did not report feeling pressurised or oppressed by what might be viewed as 'normalised' expectations, but rather they appeared to view these as their rights, just as any other non-disabled teenager would. Most parents wanted to ensure that their young people had the opportunity to get out of the house and do something meaningful, even if it was on a part time basis, rather than be isolated at home alone with a games console.

Limitations of the project

However, not all young people and families that we met over the course of the five years wanted to come to all or any of our sessions. A minority of families felt that our ideas were unrealistic, others said that, particularly in the case of the sexual health and sexuality programme, we were 'setting the boys up to fail' and that this would only bring disappointment and upset. Some families had not spoken to their young people about their impairment or its prognosis and were fearful of the impact of discussing it now (please see Chapter 6 for more about this). The use of direct payments and personal budgets can feel daunting and out of reach for some families and in these cases there is a lot of support needed to ensure families are aware of what is available and how to access any funds and resources. A very small minority of families felt uncomfortable discussing these issues.

Getting ready for work

The SEND Reforms have highlighted the need to support disabled young people into work. In our Takin' Charge workshops, young people and their families, often for the very first time, engaged in discussions about the sort of employment they would like to do in the future. We encouraged families and young people to include ideas from these discussions in their planning sessions at school and college for their Education Health and Care Plans (please see Chapter 7 for in-depth advice on EHC Plans).

We also engaged closely with the British Association of Supported Employment (BASE) to work with us on exploring barriers and solutions to getting into employment.

Initiatives such as supported internships have risen to prominence out of the SEND Reforms and are designed for learners aged

16–18 years, or for those with an EHC Plan up to the age of 24 years, who want to move into employment. Students on a supported internship are linked to a college and offered a work experience placement of approximately six months, which can be paid or unpaid. During this time, students will be supported in their placement by a job coach from the college who will mentor and assist them when required.

Alongside their time at the work placement, young people on supported internships complete a personalised study programme at college which includes the chance to study for relevant substantial qualifications. If supported internships are something that you are interested in, it is important to find out which colleges in your area offer them.

The importance of work experience

We know from the Department of Work and Pensions (2016) that doing work experience can greatly increase the chances of young people getting into employment (see Department of Health 2010). We have learned several things from supporting young people with DMD towards thinking about employment.

1. Convincing employers

First, although boys with DMD can often have the ability to work, employers can panic at the idea of a person in a wheelchair in their office, especially if there are added health and care implications. For this reason it helps to get some unpaid work if possible so that the employer can see beyond the wheelchair and realise that the young person can bring value to the workplace in the same way that any other young person might.

2. Getting skills for the workplace

Second, it enables the young people themselves to understand the expectations of the workplace and can help develop their social and professional skills, particularly if they are prone to high anxiety or social communication difficulties.

3. Finding out what you want to do

If a young person completes a work experience or supported internship that they don't like, it is not a waste of time and it doesn't mean they are not suited to the world of work. Many people have done jobs they haven't enjoyed along the way, and it's important to try things out and eliminate roles that are not for you.

4. Support from 'Access to Work' for work and work experience

In the UK there is Government support for disabled people in work called 'Access to Work' which can provide specialist equipment, personal assistance and travel. This is often referred to as the Government's best kept secret! (Sayce 2011.) Usually, Access to Work is only available to disabled people who have secured a supported internship or paid employment. Therefore, if you want to complete a work experience, you will need to think creatively about how you can get the support you need. This could involve using a PA that you may already fund from your direct payments or short breaks allowance to go to the workplace with you, or it could include less formal arrangements such as meeting a parent, friend or family member at lunchtime to help you go to the toilet or get your lunch. Ideally, you should include these costs in your Education Health and Care Plan or your support plan to ensure they will be met, but in reality you want to be able to take these opportunities when they come along. If you are doing a work experience from school or college then there should be a member of staff who can accompany you. Talk to your social worker or those in place to support you with your direct payments. As long as you are using your budget to achieve your outcomes in your plan you should be able to use this money to help with work experience costs.

The importance of good quality careers advice

Securing careers advice that can help to develop a vocational profile exploring the aptitude, skills and aspirations of the young person within their EHC Plan from the age of 14 is vital. This should be high quality personalised support from a supported employment agency with expertise in supporting disabled young people into employment, and not just a box ticking exercise with someone who has no experience of disability and employment.

Below is a snapshot of the journey of some Takin' Charge members preparing for their futures.

■ AARON, AGED 19 YEARS

Although his long-term goal was to design fashion clothing for disabled people, Aaron was keen to get experience of any workplace. A BASE member negotiated a placement with an international accountancy firm, where Aaron was expected to fulfil administrative roles such as updating data entries. Initially the company had been reluctant to take on a wheelchair user and concerned about health and safety issues, but with the help of the supported employment agency they agreed for the work experience to go ahead. From this experience, Aaron learned that he did not really want to work in office administration.

After some career profiling sessions with a supported employment agency, Aaron decided he would prefer to think about his fashion design dreams. The supported employment agency was able to broker a partnership with fashion students from a local university who were keen to find a unique project to work on. This progressed to the point of developing a proof of concept idea showing that many disabled young people want access to designer clothing and that there are fashion designers who are interested in this market. This stage of progressing an idea into a business presented challenges to Aaron because of lack of experience, skills and easy access to small business development support. However, Aaron is not down-hearted and feels that the experience has shown him that his dream is a possibility that he could pursue in the future.

At the moment, Aaron is benefiting from an unpaid supported internship with an engineering company which he is accessing through his current 19–25 placement and which includes links to the local Further Education College. Alongside their time at the work placement, young people on supported internships complete a personalised study programme which for Aaron includes the chance to improve on his English and maths grades.

During his time on Takin' Charge Aaron successfully passed his driving test and now has his licence and an adapted vehicle, which enables him to be more independent.

JACK B., AGED 17 YEARS

Jack is keen to pursue a career in scientific research. He successfully completed one week of work experience in a university research lab which has confirmed his aim to work in scientific research when he is older. Jack achieved extremely high grades in his GCSEs (formal examinations) last year and is now studying science A-levels with a view to applying to university next year. He and his family are busy attending open days at various universities and exploring the implications of Jack living away from home to study. He hopes to continue with wheelchair football in his position as goalkeeper.

SAUL, AGED 16 YEARS

Saul is keen to follow a career in Game Design. He organised work experience in a Games Design department of a London university and is now studying for a Level 3 BTEC in Software Engineering at a local Further Education college having achieved the necessary qualifications at GCSE (which took a huge amount of hard work and revision!). Saul produced a CV which he sent to independent games companies across London. He decided to tell them from the outset that he was a wheelchair user because he thought this might give him a unique selling point and would mean he wouldn't have to explain his needs later on. In fact, the company redecorated the previously unused disabled toilet in readiness for his visit! From this he has achieved a week's work experience in which he worked on several software projects and hopes to apply to other companies in order to gain valuable experience in his holidays from college. Next year Saul hopes to apply for a university course away from home in Games Design.

■ JACK E., AGED 17 YEARS

Jack is interested in Computer Aided Design and achieved a work experience placement through a partnership with a national charity and a local employer who is a major house builder. Part of his brief during the work experience was to explore what would be involved in designing accessible housing. Jack really enjoyed this experience and as a disabled person was able to bring relevant experience to the designs and make important contributions to their revisions. As a consequence of his time on work experience with them, the company have offered Jack the opportunity to start an apprenticeship. Jack is keen to pass his maths and English GCSEs before he begins this so he is currently continuing with his studies. All being well, Jack would like to start his apprenticeship next year.

■ SAM W., AGED 20 YEARS

Sam is interested in pursuing a career as a reporter and is currently studying for an undergraduate degree in journalism at the University of Winchester. To gain practical experience he has done numerous weeks of work experience with his local paper (*Southern Daily Echo*) and writes an ongoing blog[1] about issues such as being a disabled adult. In November he will be carrying out a work placement with the radio station talkSPORT in London. Alongside his studies, he enjoys his paid student ambassador role for the university. During term time, Sam lives away from home in student accommodation with carers providing full time support. He says this experience, along with travelling to America on a disability empowerment programme in 2014, has been key in developing his confidence. A place on the programme in America was secured with the support of Takin' Charge. Sam has recently returned from a week's holiday in Barcelona and intends to travel to more European cities in the future.

---

1   www.swaddersblog.wordpress.com

■ SAM B., AGED 21 YEARS

Sam gained the equivalent of three A-levels in an IT course but until recently has not felt confident enough to look for paid employment. For two years, since he finished school, he has volunteered at his local library, with the support of his local employment agency, where he supports members of the public to develop their IT skills. Often these are older people who feel left behind in this digital age. Sam has benefited from this experience and says that the role has taught him to talk to more people and not to be frightened of meeting anyone new. He recognises that the support from his local employment agency was crucial as they really helped him to find a role that he was well qualified for, and which enabled him to develop his social and emotional skills. Sam now feels much more confident and reports getting job satisfaction when he is able to explain something technical to someone he is teaching, and when they appreciate his input. In addition to volunteering at the library, Sam also volunteers with DMD Pathfinders as one of their social media team and is developing his skills in this area. Following his volunteering experiences Sam has recently decided that he is now ready to explore work placed training opportunities or even self-employment as he believes that he may have identified a gap in the market, that is, people who need 1:1 support to develop basic IT literacy and who would be prepared to pay for tuition and support.

■ DYLAN, AGED 20 YEARS

Dylan finished school at 17 and had been out of education for one year when he joined Takin' Charge. We supported him to make use of the new legislation which gives a right to all young people of 18 years to apply for an Education Health and Care Plan in their own right.

As a consequence, he was given an opportunity to undergo a full person-centred assessment. As part of this assessment he was able to articulate very clearly the life he wanted for himself as a young adult and to request the support that would be needed. Dylan was clear that he wanted the same opportunities as other 18 year olds, which meant having carers that he could choose to support him rather than his parents. He would also like to have a relationship, a job and maybe children in his life in the future.

Dylan could not read well enough to be able to be as independent as he would like. He needed personalised literacy support in his plan in order to be able to use the internet and computer. Dylan received individual literacy support as well as an IT assessment that has included voice recognition and text to speech software as part of his plan.

The special education provision within Dylan's plan includes an assessment from the British Association of Supported Employment (BASE) for a vocational career profile. He has previously had the opportunity to do some radio presentation and would quite like to pursue this as an employment opportunity. As this is part of his Education Health and Care Plan it will be reviewed on at least an annual basis with opportunities to work with a range of agencies.

Self-employment

Some of our older members were particularly interested in becoming self-employed. Self-employment offers flexibility in that people can choose their hours of work and can work from home, even if they are not able to physically manage more than a few hours work per week. However, the disadvantages of self-employment include the need to advertise yourself and have a good network of prospective clients, and the possible lack of regular work. In addition, you could miss out on what most of us enjoy about work, which is the opportunity to make new friends and colleagues.

■ MITHUN, AGED 23 YEARS

Mithun was a member of our Takin' Charge steering committee and was able to share his experiences with many young people and families. Initially, Mithun was volunteering as an ambassador for his local hospice, a national neuromuscular umbrella organisation and has now become a trustee with

DMD Pathfinders. These voluntary experiences have helped Mithun to develop his confidence as well as his public speaking skills. As a result he decided to register as a self-employed disability consultant and offers help to various organisations and charities who want advice and support around issues such as independent living and assistive technology.

Mithun secured some freelance work at a London university that runs Games Design courses as their 'Games Tester in Residence'. Students who are studying Games Design greatly benefit from working with disabled young people in order to assess the accessibility of the games they are designing. Not only has this given Mithun some income and allowed him to develop new skills, it has also served to educate a generation of young adults who are designing games that boys with DMD may enjoy playing in the future!

Mithun has also been offered work as an 'Expert by Experience' for a national social care charity providing support to disabled people and a leading UK charity for children with life-threatening and life-limiting conditions. His role is to inspect residential care homes alongside the Care Quality Commission inspectors.

In addition to this, Mithun's passion is photography and he has developed a small photography and videography business.

Summary

We hope this chapter has helped you to think about the best ways to support young people with DMD as they progress through their Transition to Adulthood. Now that the medical outlook for DMD is so much better, we look forward to hearing about the successes and challenges of the young people and families we have been privileged to get to know over the past five years. There are still far too many obstacles placed in the way for disabled young people to get the life they want, and as parents, families and professionals, it is important we pool resources and support each other. As one mother of two teenagers with DMD summed it up:

'when we got diagnosed we just thought "Oh God, our world's ended." And it hasn't – it's just they've got to do it all in a wheelchair!'

Chapter Nine

GETTING THE LIFE YOU WANT AS AN ADULT WITH DMD

John Hastie and Mark Chapman

In this chapter, Jon Hastie and Mark Chapman, who are both adults with DMD, write about their lives and how they have coped with challenges.

DR JON HASTIE

As a 36-year-old adult living with Duchenne muscular dystrophy, I can confidently say I have a fantastic life that makes me very happy. DMD has become the background noise of my life, which while I'd gladly do without, doesn't prevent me from having amazing experiences and a fulfilling life. I live independently, supported round-the-clock by carers who I employ directly. I have a PhD, make a living as a charity CEO, volunteer my time for another local disability charity, travel often, have good friends and am in a loving relationship with my boyfriend.

At the age of 16, I would never in my wildest dreams have imagined I would have such an extensive list of accomplishments and excellent quality of life at the age of 36. Indeed, back in 1997, adults living with DMD had very few prospects. With non-invasive ventilation still in its infancy, most adults living with DMD at that point passed away in their late teens and early twenties. Growing up, most of the people I knew at school with DMD had passed away.

I distinctly remember as a young teenager believing that my best hope was to live to the age of 21. I knew I had very little time to achieve anything significant. There was one young man at school, seven years older than me, who was the oldest person I knew living with DMD. After he left school, I continued to receive updates on his progress from my Mum (who knew his parents). I listened avidly as I morbidly believed he represented an upper limit of the longest life expectancy I could have, and every year he didn't die was an extra year I had to live.

I don't doubt that this sometimes painful awareness of my own mortality had a profound impact on how I viewed my life prospects. I never really thought more than two or three years ahead when considering my life's direction. At sixth form, I chose the subjects that I believed I might wish to study at university. At university, I chose the subject I believed to be the most interesting, with no consideration of the potential for entering the world of work. Had any careers adviser attempted to get me to consider employment (they didn't), I doubt I would have seriously given it any thought. To be fair, many other young people of my age may have made similar choices, but for me the justification was always on my shortened life expectancy and the need to prioritise my short-term happiness.

In some ways, focusing on short-term objectives can be the best thing we can ever do. Just take a look at all the inspiration-porn that tells us to 'live for the moment'. Certainly, treasuring what we have is an incredibly valuable life lesson for all of us. Yet in the real world, ignoring your long-term dreams and aspirations can be just as harmful as neglecting your short-term happiness.

I believe that had I known I could expect a significantly longer life than predicted, I may have taken a different path, and had a keener eye on what I wanted to achieve from a job and future career. I believe the uncertainty and lack of forward thinking slowed me down and prevented me from developing certain skills and expertise. However, in the general scheme of things I don't believe it significantly held me back. I adapted and made the most of the opportunities that arose.

As such, I don't lament the journey that I took, and don't dwell on what could have been. I simply continue moving forward. Yet in looking to inform the next generation of young adults living with DMD, I also seek to learn from my past. I see young adults with DMD planning for the future now and recognise that when their own preconceptions are challenged, we see budding entrepreneurs and individuals with incredible potential emerge. That's why I encourage every young man living with DMD to consider a future where at age 50, they reflect back on their lives and what they have done.

Going to university

At the age of 18, I had received excellent grades both at A-level and GCSE level, two years previously. I was a diligent student, had an excellent circle of friends with whom I socialised both in and out of school, played wheelchair hockey regularly and had been in a relationship with my girlfriend for one year. Having seen my brother go to Bristol University three years previously, with my strong academic record university seemed like the obvious choice. I selected the university I wished to attend based on a range of different academic and disability-related criteria. It had to be within three hours travelling distance of my parents, had to have a good academic programme, and had to offer the support necessary for me to live in university halls.

Living at university was never really in question. Having seen how my brother thrived and the fantastic friends that he made (who he remains very close to this day), I knew that living away from home in halls was an integral part of the whole university experience that I couldn't afford to miss. This is perhaps one of the best decisions I have ever made and one of the best pieces of advice I could give to anyone considering university. The academic education is just one aspect of what university has to offer. It also offers powerful social and practical education, opening you up to new experiences, new cultures and giving you the opportunity to make friends for life.

That's not to say these awesome experiences happen overnight or with little effort. Moving away from home takes its toll on everyone, and this is even more true for those of us with DMD, who have often relied on parents to manage every aspect of our care. Making friends can be easier for some than others, and it takes courage and effort to put yourself out there and initiate conversations and build friendships over time. A wobble or two is to be expected, and at some point or other you will be tempted to throw in the towel and give up. Recognising this, and the fact that every new student is in the same position, can be helpful in finding the will to persevere.

A key part of my choice of university was to select a place where my accessible room was integrated into the wider student population. This was important to me as I have always been a strong believer in integration rather than segregation. The university experience was a vital one in helping me to meet and understand people from a wide variety of backgrounds. I believe that having made friends at school with both disabled and non-disabled people, I was in a better position to relate with and interact socially with non-disabled students that I lived with.

At a fully accessible campus university, I was able to engage in student life to the full, and very rarely found that having DMD significantly affected my experience. I engaged in fairly typical student behaviour including being involved in pranks, parties and sometimes excessive drinking, but also the more responsible side of academic studies and student politics. Occasionally, the real world would penetrate the campus bubble, as friends went to inaccessible nightclubs, or when they were forced to move off campus to inaccessible houses (only being allowed to live on campus for one year compared to my permanent residence for the duration of my studies). All in all, I don't think I fared too badly out of the deal. I never got to experience life in a no-holds barred student house, yet I did get to enjoy the benefits of campus life with a new tranche of flatmates every year.

The freedom provided by the fully accessible environment and the diverse social life I experienced made it easy to continue the university lifestyle. As such, with good grades I was able to progress to a Master's degree and then a PhD over the eight years that I attended. The university years were the best of my life, and I don't believe I would choose any differently if I was cast back to that time now. Yet beneath this seemingly obvious choice was a more problematic context. In choosing to stay at university, I was not choosing between two possible options. At the time, the university option seemed the only viable one. I didn't know of anyone living with DMD who had ever successfully navigated the fields of work or the 'real world' and made a great success of it. It seemed a scary prospect and one that could likely lead me to living at home with my parents with no meaningful activity to engage in. All too often, and still to this day, that is exactly what happens for people with DMD leaving school or college.

Getting employment

In 2008, having moved back home with my parents, I was keen to enter the world of work and applied for a range of jobs including academic posts. As someone who had never applied for a job before, I was quickly disheartened by the limited response to my few applications. While now I appreciate the tough competition for jobs and the fact that my limited number of applications was never going to be sufficient, at the time I questioned whether I would ever be able to find a job that met my needs and interests.

Having recently gained a PhD, what I knew for certain was that I couldn't sit at home doing nothing beyond playing computer games. I took on a volunteering role at a local disability organisation, reviewing entertainment venues and restaurants for their accessibility to disabled people. While not especially challenging, it opened me up to a new network of friends and amazing people, united in a mission to improve the local area for disabled people. It also allowed me to work alongside staff in a professional office environment and gave me the flexibility to take initiative and contribute more than was initially expected in the volunteer role. This placed me in an excellent position to take advantage of a job-share opportunity at the organisation when it came up six months later.

It was this organisation, then called the Brighton and Hove Federation of Disabled People (now Possability People), that was instrumental in supporting me to enter the world of work, encouraging me to make the most of the opportunity and giving me the support I needed to become a paid employee. This offered me an excellent challenge, and the room to grow and change roles. It significantly developed my transferable skills as well as building confidence in my own ability, which allowed me to progress to more demanding jobs in other organisations. Having at times not expected to work at all, I certainly didn't in my younger years believe that I would be able to move between different organisations and be selective in the jobs that I did, rather than taking whatever I could get. By the way, I still play computer games.

In hindsight, it is somewhat remarkable that, with a PhD, I was so lacking in confidence and awareness of my own skills and potential that I almost didn't apply for that first job. It took the encouragement of the amazing CEO to even apply. Evidently, she had a keen eye for potential because I certainly thrived in that environment. Looking back on my life prior to that point, I believe that I missed opportunities to learn about my own capabilities and skills. Prior to leaving college, I was never able to gain significant work experience, as many employers back then simply didn't want the difficulties involved in having a disabled trainee in the workplace. Ever since, I had stuck to academia and saw the real world of work as an arena that my health and care needs would never allow me to enter. In many ways, this bad experience at college and the insight it had given me into workplace barriers was completely disabling for a long period of time. It led me and my parents to internalise the barriers imposed by employers (such as inaccessible workplaces or inflexible working hours) as my own personal lack of capability as an adult living with DMD. This was somewhat self-reinforcing as my parents, keen I was not disappointed by the lack of opportunity, suggested that I should prepare myself for the fact that perhaps volunteering was all I could do. It has taken many years of self-realisation and the excellent support provided by a number of employers to make me realise that I can work and have a lot to offer, if the employer is supportive.

Coping with health challenges

As previously stated, I consider DMD to be the background noise my life. That's not to say it does not have a profound impact on the way I live my life. However, over time I have learnt how to live with it, how to manage the consequences of the condition, and how to minimise the disruptive impact it can have. I take a fairly scientific and analytical approach to the condition, paying attention to small changes and experimenting with different solutions. For example, having experienced significant chewing and swallowing problems as well as weight loss, irritable bowel and constipation, I have by a process of elimination and experimentation identified an appropriate diet which I seek to maintain. Recognising the importance of preventing coughs, colds and chest infections, I have an elaborate system of herbal remedies, cold-prevention sprays, and prophylactic antibiotics to avoid these from disrupting my life. I have a keen awareness of how I'm feeling at any time and adapt appropriately, getting sufficient rest and adapting my work schedule around my needs. I manage my own care and support so I can be confident that I am supported by reliable people, allowing me to promptly deal with any employment issues or unsatisfactory performance by care staff, and keep everything functioning efficiently.

Securing a care package

At the age of 18, I benefited from the Independent Living Fund, which contributed a top-up amount to my social care package provided by my local Adult Social Care team (social services). Social services are focused on meeting the most basic personal care needs of a large population; while they have a legal duty to meet someone's care needs, support has always been inadequate to allow someone to live an independent life. The Independent Living Fund was a national fund set up to compensate for this inadequacy. I was lucky enough to benefit from this until 2014, when I transitioned to a Continuing Healthcare (CHC) package funded exclusively by the NHS, a generous but incredibly difficult programme to qualify for which is only open to people with the most complex needs. The Independent Living Fund was subsequently closed in 2015. What this means is that adults with DMD now have to rely on far less support, prompting extensive battles with social services to obtain limited care.

At university, I received a package of care from social services, the Independent Living Fund and the Disabled Students Allowance. This was not sufficient to pay for qualified carers, and instead required me to use a volunteer agency. Volunteers from all over the world applied to this agency to engage in meaningful nine-month volunteering placements. The quality of care was quite limited, with many volunteers being 18-year-olds with no care experience whatsoever. Yet since I had relatively basic needs at this point, the care was sufficient and it allowed me to meet some amazing people with very diverse backgrounds. While I was fairly independent, as live-in carers who lived above me in student halls, the volunteers were always on hand should I require them.

Moving back from university to my parents' home, we negotiated with social services to continue this volunteer-based care package, with an increased contribution as I no longer received the Disabled Students Allowance. Given the fact I had moved in with my parents, there was a clear expectation by social services that my parents would provide the bulk of my care. My parents and I were keen that this did not happen, as after seven years of living independently at university we felt this would be a regressive step. The only way to prevent this was for my parents to clearly and unequivocally state to social services that they were unwilling to provide any of my care. Thankfully, they could not be forced to do so, meaning the duty remained with social services to meet my needs. Social services refused but, after a campaign that caused headlines in two local TV stations, the NHS stepped in to make up the shortfall.

In 2014, I had a similarly drawn out, yet eventually successful, fight for funding, as I was again assessed and refused for the NHS Continuing Healthcare programme. For now, my needs are fully met by an extensive, 24/7, care package. I certainly feel lucky compared to others who are still struggling, but know I would never be in this position had I not fought tooth and nail for support.

The care support I receive has been and continues to be an absolutely fundamental part of what allows me to have a good quality of life as an adult living with DMD. Most importantly, it is the flexibility of my care package that enabled me to have such a positive university experience, and to realise my aspirations since. While our social care and health system continues to relentlessly focus on medical problems and personal care needs, it is the support I have received in meeting my *social* needs that has been most important in securing my quality of life. Most often, this support has only been available as a consequence of my personal care needs. In my present situation, for example, it is only my dependence on my ventilator and the need to be accompanied 24/7 to prevent respiratory failure that has ensured I have round-the-clock care, which allows me to visit friends and family and engage extensively in community activity. For many other adults with other conditions without such high personal care needs, they can be lucky to receive sufficient support to get out of the house once a week.

Friends, relationships and sexuality

Social isolation is a huge risk for all disabled adults, and in particular adults living with DMD, who often cannot rely on the long-standing friendships that older adults might. On leaving school, college or university, we are presented with a situation where our ability to socialise is significantly constrained, at a time when friendships naturally drift apart due to life getting in the way. Whether due to the lack of care support, or the fact that many adult friendships are built through work, visiting people in their often inaccessible homes or meeting up in inaccessible venues, adults with DMD are at a significant disadvantage when it comes to making new friends. I have often felt this frustration, when groups I have become involved with invite me to a venue I cannot enter. Meanwhile existing friends have become increasingly separated, often requiring extensive travel to maintain friendships.

It's an area that continues to challenge and frustrate me personally, and for many, can have very real health complications such as depression and other mental health problems. Yet, mind-bogglingly, it is rarely meaningfully included in support and care plans when designing support packages. Thankfully, my involvement in work and volunteering with community organisations has provided me with opportunities to meet new friends, and has been a remarkable source of support.

The last and most recent progress I've made in securing the life I want is in the area of sexuality and relationships. This was one aspect of my happiness that has always eluded me and has been significantly complicated by my sexuality as a gay disabled man. Throughout adulthood I have had carers very intimately involved in every aspect of my life, and privacy has been incredibly hard to come by. At university, while many of the volunteers who supported me were fantastic, I had no opportunity to make sure they would support how I wanted to live my life, and no real privacy from them. Here I was, a young gay man struggling with his identity and feeling a heavy dose of guilt for being attracted to other men. While I watched others join LGBT student clubs I fretted about how I could possibly do that without my carers finding out.

As a consequence, I never felt capable of coming out in my younger years. It's telling that it was only at the age of 30, after finally moving into my own flat to live independently and recruiting my own Personal Assistants (PAs) to support me with care, that I felt able to actually be myself and came out. At that point, I was finally in a position where I could recruit those PAs I felt would be supportive of my life choices.

Alongside the struggles of recognising my sexuality came the increasingly difficult struggle with my own self-image and self esteem, as DMD increasingly took a physical toll on my body. Although this had been progressing all my life, a step-change occurred when I started to use my ventilator more during the daytime, wearing an ugly, obstructive mask over my face. Perversely, this occurred just at the time I felt confident in expressing my sexuality, and knocked me back significantly. It took me quite a long time to feel comfortable wearing it in public. Although on the whole, people still treated me the same, I definitely encountered more stares from people wondering what on earth this mask was. Although I gained confidence and became comfortable with the mask in public, many questions wouldn't stop playing in my head such as 'how will anyone find me attractive?', 'how can I even kiss anyone now?'

During this period my approach to online dating was sporadic. I'd get inspired by a positive story of someone with DMD finding love and have a flurry of activity, often with minimal response, at which point I'd give up. Online dating felt like signing up to be repeatedly punched in the face. Over the course of three or four years of sporadic online activity there were maybe three or four people who seemed genuinely interested, yet I felt no attraction to them. My lack of luck attracting others didn't make me so desperate that my preferences didn't matter.

During 2013 I started using a new ventilator which I operated via a mouthpiece rather than a mask over my face. This relatively small change took a lot of getting used to, but was transformative in how I viewed my own attractiveness. It gave me a real boost. And then, the day before my 35th birthday, one of these bursts of online dating activity sparked a conversation with a guy where the attractiveness and chemistry were clear and mutual. We chatted for a few months, and I crossed new boundaries into Skype-dating, which was not without its share of physical challenges. Since then we have met up in person several times and embarked on an emotional journey I never believed I would ever get to take.

Without a doubt, love has been the hardest thing to find in my life so far. I don't want to be dismissed as a hopeless romantic by saying that everyone with DMD can find a suitable partner, because the harsh reality is that the challenges are immense. But equally it could happen – and for me, even the remotest possibility felt worth pursuing.

And finally

In terms of my own experience, I would urge people to challenge the limited assumptions others may have of them, as well as their own assumptions and expectations of society around them. Be curious about everything and even if you believe something might be impossible, make sure you thoroughly research and explore the problem and potential solutions before you give up on it. There are enough genuine barriers out there that we don't need to be assuming new ones that might not be real.

MARK CHAPMAN

I am a 47-year-old adult living with DMD in Edinburgh. As you have probably discovered from reading this book, young people with DMD are all individual, and my story is very different from Jon's in many ways, and similar in others. I currently live in my own flat, with 24-hour PA support.

Early life

I grew up in a very rural area of Berwickshire and attended the local village school which only had 11 pupils. After regular spates of falling over, I was diagnosed with DMD at the age of 6 years. My parents were told that I was not likely to live into adulthood. I started using a wheelchair at the age of 10 years and so the most suitable secondary school for me was a special school an hour away from home in Edinburgh, which had a residential unit for children with physical impairments. Although I missed my parents and my two brothers terribly to begin with, I met some good friends who I still regularly socialise with now. However, I think my living away from home was very difficult for my parents in many ways, and it also meant that I lost local friends. Also, I think many young people in the special school missed out on education and getting academic qualifications because assumptions were made about people's ability because they were disabled. For example, I had a good friend who had cerebral palsy and was very clever but whose aspirations were not taken seriously because of his impairment.

After school

After school I returned home, but the choices of what to do next were very limited there and the local college did not offer any courses that I was interested in following. I was very keen to start a Graphic Design course in Edinburgh and to live independently like other young adults my age. However, this life would have to be funded from the local authority. As most of you know, trying to get support and resources can be an extremely difficult and stressful process. It took over a year of fighting to secure adequate funding for the specialist support and accommodation necessary for me to attend Further Education College. My local MP at the time played a crucial role in supporting my case with the local suthority. If you're having a particularly difficult issue I would encourage you to contact your MP. Local authorities, for example, don't like receiving letters from MPs so it can really help your cause.

Eventually, I managed to move into a shared flat in a brand new supported, independent living accommodation in Edinburgh. I was able to follow a course that interested me with extra support at college from a Community Service volunteer, and I completed a Higher National Diploma in Illustration and Media Design in 1994. Like most students I had a very active social life involving many pubs, clubs and quite a few parties!

Health issues and respiration

After college, my health deteriorated and at the age of 24 I wasn't really sure I would survive much longer. I had been told that I would be lucky to reach the age of 25 years and that I should expect these sort of health problems. At this time I was sharing the flat with my girlfriend, Corinna, who I had met at school. I kept getting chest infections and I was grumpy and tired, not eating very well and probably a bit of a nightmare to live with! I had almost given up speaking as it was such an effort to string a sentence together. One of my old school friends with DMD who had recently got married had been given a tracheostomy as an emergency procedure due to respiratory failure. This seemed to have helped him enormously and this inspired me to explore this option before it became an emergency. Thanks to a very committed doctor at the Edinburgh Western General Hospital, I had a tracheostomy in September 1996. This felt like a very big step beforehand, as I knew that there were risks involved in having this procedure. However, my health challenges reduced massively from the moment that it was done.

After a few months' recovery and adjustment I suddenly had a new lease of life. I had more energy, it was easier to talk, my appetite improved dramatically and, most importantly, secretions could be easily suctioned from my lungs through the tracheostomy, significantly reducing chest infections. I only found out afterwards that respiration problems can cause a whole host of problems such as lack of appetite, irritability and general inertia. It is important to look out for these signs as well as loud snoring or episodes of not breathing during the night and make sure you ask for regular sleep studies. These can identify whether you are getting a build-up of carbon dioxide in your body which is very harmful.

Surprisingly, living with a tracheostomy has not been too difficult. I've adapted very well. With training and back up from an NHS community team, my PAs are able to carry out procedures for my life support without much problem. As long as you are clear and organised, PAs can deal well with the responsibility.

Developing the skills to live independently

This determination of mine has certainly played a part in the independent life I live today. Fighting for everything was the reality; it still is. Housing, equipment, PAs, good health, mobility, relationship, activities and so on. Nothing comes easily. Nonetheless, the value in being responsible for yourself and in control of your life cannot be underestimated! It's a fantastic feeling. With many of us living well into adulthood it is more important than ever we develop our own lives. Our parents cannot support us indefinitely; they have concerns about getting older and ill in the future. Although letting go can be a struggle for parents, there is security with us living independent lives with support. At the moment, I employ five PAs who provide 24-hour care for me on a rota system. Of course, achieving this independence involves many battles – some you'll win, some you'll lose – and more often than not you'll accept a compromise. Since the cuts, it is becoming more and more difficult for carers to live on the wages we give them, and this is very worrying both for them and for disabled people who can only live independently if this support is available.

Of course, living independently does bring with it many responsibilities. There are meals to plan, bills to pay and shopping to be done. PAs need to be recruited and managed like any other employee and they need contracts, training and wages every month. If you have a car or van, this needs insuring and servicing. Pets need feeding and taking to the vet. All of this needs to be thought about, planned for and budgeted. If you're clear about how you spend the funding and keep within budget then the funder is less likely to question anything.

Employment, voluntary work and social life

Although I haven't worked in a paid role, I have kept busy and fulfilled through a variety of voluntary roles. I would urge people to think seriously about what they want to do as a career and make sure the support you need is in place. A job, whether it's paid or voluntary, gives you the chance to meet new people and have a social life. It gets you out of the house and doing something interesting and valuable.

Now that adults with DMD are living longer it is crucial that your aspirations are discussed and planned for or they just won't happen. When I was growing up, my future plans were the 'elephant in the room' – nobody asked me what I wanted to do, because they didn't think I'd be alive. And here I am at 46 years old!

My friends are a very important part of my life and I do feel that having an active social life keeps you sane. We meet up at least once a week for a drink or to go to the cinema, and when the Edinburgh Festival is on I'm never home! I have strong political beliefs and have been on a lot of marches in my time such as the Anti-Poll Tax demonstration in the late 1980s and marches for Scottish devolution. These days a lot of my time is focused on exploring best ways to support the rights of disabled people, and particularly those with DMD.

For many years, I was the chair of the Scottish Muscle Group and I am still an active member of the Cross Party Group for Muscular Dystrophy in the Scottish Parliament. From 2011 to 2016 I was a steering committee member of Action D Takin' Charge's Transition to Adulthood project, along with Jon Hastie, where we supported the strategic direction of the project and facilitated workshops and seminars with young people with DMD and their families.

Plans for the future

From supporting the Takin' Charge steering committee, Jon and I have gone on to set up the first user-led organisation for people with DMD called DMD Pathfinders. We are incredibly excited about this and feel that for the first time we are able to give voice to people who live with DMD, rather than have decisions about campaigns or funding made for us by those who do not live with our challenges or insights. This year we will be hosting our first conference and have many plans to ensure that adults with DMD are not forgotten in research, have access to excellent care and the chance to live the best life possible.

Biographies of Contributors

Dr Janet Hoskin is a Senior Lecturer at the Cass School of Education and Communities, University of East London, where she teaches on undergraduate and postgraduate Special Education programmes. In 2001, when their son Saul was diagnosed with DMD, Janet co-founded the national charity Action Duchenne with Nick Catlin, and from 2008 to 2011 she ran Action Duchenne's lottery funded 'Include Duchenne' project which worked with over 60 children with DMD, their families and schools across the UK and which won the 2011 National Lottery Education Award. From 2011 to 2016 Janet co-managed the 'Takin' Charge' Transition to Adulthood project working with 80 young people with DMD aged 14–19 years and their families. In 2013–2014, Janet also managed a Leadership Programme for young adults with DMD for Decipha CIC, which was funded by the Department for Education. She is currently researching the impact of the SEND Reforms on young people with life-limiting impairments, their families and schools.

Dr Kate Maresh is a Specialty Doctor in Neurology at the Royal Free Hospital in London, and a Clinical Research Fellow in Professor Muntoni's research group at the Dubowitz Neuromuscular Centre, Great Ormond Street Institute of Child Health, University College London. She is a study doctor for several clinical trials in DMD at Great Ormond Street Hospital, and is undertaking research into how the brain is affected in DMD.

Professor Francesco Muntoni is a Paediatric Neurologist with a strong clinical and academic interest in childhood neuromuscular disorders. He leads the Dubowitz Neuromuscular Centre at the Great Ormond Street Institute of Child Health, University College London.

Since the early 1990s he has been involved in studies on the correlation between genotype and phenotype in Duchenne and Becker muscular dystrophy and in X-linked dilated cardiomyopathy. In the last decade he has been involved in translational research aspects and clinical trials for Duchenne muscular dystrophy. He edited two monographs on Duchenne muscular dystrophy with Professor Alan Emery, and has co-authored more than 100 peer reviewed manuscripts on Duchenne over the last 30 years.

Veronica Hinton, PhD is an Associate Professor of Neuropsychology in the G.H. Sergievsky Center and Department of Neurology at Columbia University. She researches the cognitive and behavioral characteristics of different pediatric disorders and also runs the Pediatric Neuropsychology clinical service in Child Neurology at Columbia University Medical Center. Dr Hinton has had the pleasure of working with children with dystrophinopathies for twenty years.

Lianne Abbott and Victoria Selby have worked as physiotherapists in the neuromuscular team at Great Ormond Street Hospital (GOSH) and Institute of Child Health (ICH) in London for five and eight years respectively. Both have extensive paediatric neuromuscular experience within the clinical and research field. They are passionate about physiotherapy and education and are proactive in sharing knowledge and helping continued progression in the management and treatment of neuromuscular conditions.

David J. Schonfeld MD, FAAP is a developmental-behavioral pediatrician and Professor of Practice in the Suzanne Dworak-Peck School of Social Work and Pediatrics at the University of Southern California (USC) and Children's Hospital Los Angeles. He has conducted research on children's understanding of illness, written and evaluated elementary school curricula on HIV/AIDS and cancer, published research articles and book chapters on the topic, and spoken to parent and professional audiences on how to help children understand and adjust to DMD.

James Poysky, PhD, is a clinical psychologist and pediatric neuropsychologist who is recognised as an expert in the learning, emotional, and behavioral challenges associated with Duchenne muscular dystrophy. He holds a faculty position of Clinical Assistant

Professor at Baylor College of Medicine and also works in private practice. Dr. Poysky lives with his family in Katy, Texas, a suburb of the greater Houston area. He enjoys travelling, cooking and playing soccer. He is married and has two children, including a 14-year-old son with DMD.

Nick Catlin is a Special Educational Needs and Disability (SEND) Advisory Teacher and is currently developing the RoadMap for Life Programme for Decipha CIC to support young people and their families living with Duchenne muscular dystrophy.

Nick was a founding member and CEO of the Charity Action Duchenne. Action Duchenne led the development of new genetic treatments for Duchenne Muscular Dystrophy and new programmes to support the assessment and intervention for those young people with learning and behaviour problems. He has a son who is living with Duchenne muscular dystrophy. Nick developed the first national online Clinical Trial Registry for Duchenne muscular dystrophy.

Nick has been a Special Educational Needs Coordinator (SENCO) in an East London Secondary School and the Deputy Head of a Pupil Referral Unit. He has worked with children with SEND for over 30 years, including children with complex and severe communication difficulties, and has a special interest in assessing and offering support to young people with emotional and behaviour difficulties.

Celine Barry is an independent Special Educational Needs and Disability (SEND) consultant in the UK, working with Special Needs Coordinators in schools as well as parents, young people and adults affected by Duchenne. Celine achieved a successful career as a teacher and manager in a range of specialist and mainstream settings including as an Assistant Headteacher for Inclusion in a mainstream secondary school, where she managed provision for pupils with complex medical, physical, learning and behaviour needs. She has had a professional interest in Transition and brought this to the role of co-managing Action Duchenne's successful Takin' Charge project with Janet Hoskin from 2011 to 2016. Celine has a nephew with Duchenne who is 24 years old.

Dr Jon Hastie is 36 and an adult living with Duchenne muscular dystrophy. He is also CEO of DMD Pathfinders, a user-led organisation of adults living with Duchenne which provides advice, guidance and support for other teenagers and adults living with the condition. Jon is a key patient advocate and campaigner and produced the 2012 documentary *A Life Worth Living: Pushing the Limits of Duchenne*, which followed his journey around the UK and Europe to meet other adults living with DMD. In 2014 he co-founded DMD Pathfinders with Mark Chapman, a fellow adult with DMD.

Jon lives independently in his own flat in Shoreham by Sea, supported by a team of personal assistants who provide round-the-clock care. He was awarded a PhD in government in 2008 and has since worked in two separate disability charities and as a political assistant at a City Council before taking up his role at DMD Pathfinders.

Mark Chapman receives 24/7 tracheostomy ventilation and, aged 47, is one of the eldest in the UK living with Duchenne muscular dystrophy. He's lived independently in Edinburgh for over 25 years and is supported by employing his own team of Personal Assistants. As co-founder and chair of DMD Pathfinders he's actively committed to campaigning for improved care and support for those with Duchenne and similar conditions.

References

Introduction

Abbott, D., Carpenter, J. and Bushby, K. (2012) 'Transition to Adulthood for Young Men with Duchenne Muscular Dystrophy : research from the UK'. *Neuromuscular Disorders*, 22, 445–6.

Astrea, G., Pecini, C., Gasperini, F. *et al.* (2015) 'Reading impairment in Duchenne muscular dystrophy: A pilot study to investigate similarities and differences with developmental dyslexia.' *Research in Developmental Disabilities 45–46*, 1681–1677.

Billard, C., Gillet, P., Barthez, M., Hommet, C. and Bertrand, P. (1998) 'Reading ability and processing in Duchenne muscular dystrophy and spinal muscular atrophy.' *Developmental Medicine and Child Neurology 40*, 1, 12–20.

Bushby, K., Finkel, R., Birnkrant, D.J., Case, L.E. *et al.* (2010) 'DMD Care Considerations Working Group. Diagnosis and management of Duchenne Muscular Dystrophy, Part 1: Diagnosis, and pharmacological and psychosocial management.' *Lancet Neurology 9*, 1, 404–408.

Department for Education and Department of Health (2015) Special Educational Needs and Disability Code of Practice 0 to 25 years. Available at www.gov. uk/government/publications/send-code-of-practice-0-to-25, accessed on 07 July 2017.

Eagle, M., Bourke, J., Bullock, R., Gibson, M. *et al.* (2007) 'Managing Duchenne muscular dystrophy – the additive effect of spinal surgery and home nocturnal ventilation in improving survival.' *Neuromuscular Disorders 17*, 470–475.

Hendriksen, J.G. and Vles, J.S. (2008) 'Are males with Duchenne muscular dystrophy at risk for reading disabilities?' *Pediatric Neurology 2008*, 34, 296–300.

Hinton, V.J., De Vivo, D.C., Fee, R.., Goldstein, E. and Stern, Y. (2004) 'Investigation of poor academic achievement in children with Duchenne Muscular Dystrophy.' *Learning Disabilities Research and Practice 19*, 3, 146–154.

Landfeldt, E., Lindgren, P., Bell, C.F., Guglieri, M., Straub, V., Lochmuller, H. and Bushby, K (2015) 'Health-related quality of life in patients with Duchenne muscular dystrophy: A multinational, cross-sectional study.' *Developmental Medicine and Child Neurology 58*, 5, 508–515.

Leibowitz, D. and Dubowitz, V. (1981) 'Intellect and behaviour in Duchenne Muscular Dystrophy.' *Developmental Medicine and Child Neurology 23*, 6, 577–590.

Rahbek, J., Werge, B., Madsen, A., Fynbo, C., Steffensen, B. and Jeppesen, J. (2005) 'Adult life with Duchenne muscular dystrophy: Observations among an emerging and unforeseen patient population.' *Paediatric Rehabilitation 8*, 1, 17–28.

Thomas, C. (1999) *Experiencing and Understanding Disability.* Buckingham: Open University Press.

Chapter 1

Aartsma-Rus, A., Van Deutekom, J.C., Fokkema, I.F., Van Ommen, G.J. and Den Dunnen, J.T. (2006) 'Entries in the Leiden Duchenne muscular dystrophy mutation database: An overview of mutation types and paradoxical cases that confirm the reading-frame rule.' *Muscle and Nerve 34*, 2, 135–144.

Anderson, J.L., Head, S.I. and Morley, J.W. (2012) 'Duchenne Muscular Dystrophy and Brain Function'. In Dr Madhuri Hedge (ed.) InTech. Available at www.intechopen.com/books/muscular-dystrophy/brain-function-in-duchenne-muscular-dystrophy, accessed on 7 December 2016

Astrea, G., Pecini, C., Gasperini, F. *et al.* (2015) 'Reading impairment in Duchenne muscular dystrophy: A pilot study to investigate similarities and differences with developmental dyslexia.' *Research into Developmental Disabilities 45–46*, 168–177.

Banihani, R., Smile, S., Yoon, G. *et al.* (2015) 'Cognitive and neurobehavioral profile in boys with Duchenne muscular dystrophy.' *Journal of Child Neurology 30*, 11, 1472–1482.

Bechara, A., Damasio, H. and Damasio, A.R. (2003) 'Role of the amygdala in decision-making.' *Annals of the New York Academy of Sciences 985*, 356–369.

Billard, C., Gillet, P., Signoret, J.L. *et al.* (1992) 'Cognitive functions in Duchenne muscular dystrophy: A reappraisal and comparison with spinal muscular atrophy.' *Neuromuscular Disorders 2*, 5–6, 371–378.

Billard, C., Gillet, P., Barthez, M., Hommet, C. and Bertrand, P. (1998) 'Reading ability and processing in Duchenne muscular dystrophy and spinal muscular atrophy.' *Developmental Medicine and Child Neurology 40*, 1, 12–20.

Blackburn, C. and Spencer N. (2012) 'Children with Neurodevelopmental disabilities.' In: Department of Health Annual Report of the Chief Medical Officer 2012, Our Children Deserve Better: Prevention Pays.

Brauner, C.B. and Stephens, C.B. (2006) 'Estimating the prevalence of early childhood serious emotional/behavioral disorders: Challenges and recommendations.' *Public Health Reports 121*, 3, 303–310.

Buckner, R.L. (2013) 'The cerebellum and cognitive function: 25 years of insight from anatomy and neuroimaging.' *Neuron 80*, 3, 807–815.

Cartwright-Hatton, S., McNicol, K. and Doubleday, E. (2006) 'Anxiety in a neglected population: Prevalence of anxiety disorders in pre-adolescent children.' *Clinical Psychology Review 26*, 7, 817–833.

Caspers-Conway, K., Mathews, K.D., Paramsothy, P. *et al.* (2015) 'Neurobehavioral concerns among males with dystrophinopathy using population-based surveillance data from the Muscular Dystrophy Surveillance, Tracking, and Research Network.' *Journal of Developmental and Behavioral Pediatrics 36*, 6, 455–463.

Chaussenot, R., Edeline, J.M., Le Bec, B., El Massioui, N., Laroche, S. and Vaillend, C. (2015) 'Cognitive dysfunction in the dystrophin-deficient mouse model of Duchenne muscular dystrophy: A reappraisal from sensory to executive processes.' *Neurobiology of Learning and Memory 124*, 111–122.

Costello, E.J., Mustillo, S., Erkanli, A., Keeler, G. and Angold, A. (2003) 'Prevalence and development of psychiatric disorders in childhood and adolescence.' *Archives of General Psychiatry 60*, 8, 837–844.

Cotton, S., Voudouris, N.J. and Greenwood, K.M. (2001) 'Intelligence and Duchenne muscular dystrophy: Full-scale, verbal, and performance intelligence quotients.' *Developmental Medicine and Child Neurology 43*, 7, 497–501.

Cowan, L.D. (2002) 'The epidemiology of the epilepsies in children.' *Mental Retardation and Developmental Disabilities Research Reviews 8*, 3, 171–181.

Cyrulnik, S.E., Fee, R.J., De Vivo, D.C., Goldstein, E. and Hinton, V.J. (2007) 'Delayed developmental language milestones in children with Duchenne's muscular dystrophy.' *The Journal of Pediatrics 150*, 5, 474–478.

Darke, J., Bushby, K., Le Couteur, A. and McConachie, H. (2006) 'Survey of behaviour problems in children with neuromuscular diseases.' *European Journal of Paediatric Neurology: EJPN: Official Journal of the European Paediatric Neurology Society 10*, 3, 129–134.

Donders, J. and Taneja, C. (2009) 'Neurobehavioral characteristics of children with Duchenne muscular dystrophy.' *Child Neuropsychology: A Journal on Normal and Abnormal Development in Childhood and Adolescence 15*, 3, 295–304.

Doorenweerd, N., Straathof, C.S., Dumas, E.M. *et al.* (2014) 'Reduced cerebral gray matter and altered white matter in boys with Duchenne muscular dystrophy.' *Annals of Neurology 76*, 3, 403–411.

Dubowitz, V. and Crome, L. (1969) 'The central nervous system in Duchenne muscular dystrophy.' *Brain: A Journal of Neurology 92*, 4, 805–808.

Eldevik, S., Jahr, E., Eikeseth, S., Hastings, R.P. and Hughes, C.J. (2010) 'Cognitive and adaptive behavior outcomes of behavioral intervention for young children with intellectual disability.' [Erratum appears in Behaviour Modification. 2010 Mar;34(2):191-2]. *Behaiour Modification 34*, 1, 16–34.

Emery, A.E.H., Muntoni, F. and Quinlivan, R. (2015) 'Involvement of tissues other than skeletal muscle.' *Duchenne Muscular Dystrophy* (4th edition). Oxford: Oxford University Press.

Etemadifar, M. and Molaei, S. (2004) 'Epilepsy in boys with Duchenne Muscular Dystrophy.' *Journal of Research in Medical Sciences 9*, 3, 116–119.

Fombonne, E. (2003) 'Epidemiological surveys of autism and other pervasive developmental disorders: An update.' *Journal of Autism and Developmental Disorders 33*, 4, 365–382.

Goodnough, C.L., Gao, Y., Li, X. *et al.* (2014) 'Lack of dystrophin results in abnormal cerebral diffusion and perfusion in vivo.' *Neuroimage 102 Pt 2*, 809–816.

Goodwin, F., Muntoni, F. and Dubowitz, V. (1997) 'Epilepsy in Duchenne and Becker muscular dystrophies.' *European Journal of Paediatric Neurology: EJPN: Official Journal of the European Paediatric Neurology Society 1*, 4, 115–119.

Goyenvalle, A., Griffith, G., Babbs, A. *et al.* (2015) 'Functional correction in mouse models of muscular dystrophy using exon-skipping tricyclo-DNA oligomers.' *Nature Medicine 21*, 3, 270–275.

Green, H., Meltzer, H., Ford, T. and Goodman, R. (2005) 'Mental health of children and young people in Great Britain, 2004. A survey carried out by the Office for National Statistics on behalf of the Department of Health and the Scottish Executive.' Basingstoke: Palgrave Macmillan.

Groenewegen, H.J. and Uylings, H.B.M. (2000) 'The Prefrontal Cortex and the Integration of Sensory, Limbic and Autonomic Information.' In H.B.M. Uylings, J.P.C De Bruin, M.G.E. Feenstra and C.M.A Pennartz (eds) *Progress in Brain Research*. Amsterdam, Netherlands: Elsevier.

Guralnick, M.J. (2016) 'Early intervention for children with intellectual disabilities: An update.' *Journal of Applied Research in Intellectual Disabilities 13*, 13.

Hendriksen, J.G. and Vles, J.S. (2008) 'Neuropsychiatric disorders in males with duchenne muscular dystrophy: Frequency rate of attention-deficit hyperactivity disorder (ADHD), autism spectrum disorder, and obsessive-compulsive disorder.' *Journal of Child Neurology 23*, 5, 477–481.

Hendriksen, R.G., Hoogland, G., Schipper, S., Hendriksen, J.G., Vles, J.S. and Aalbers, M.W. (2015) 'A possible role of dystrophin in neuronal excitability: A review of the current literature.' *Neuroscience and Biobehavioral Reviews 51*, 255–262.

Hendriksen, R.G.F., Schipper, S., Hoogland, G. *et al.* (2016) 'Dystrophin distribution and expression in human and experimental temporal lobe epilepsy.' *Frontiers in Cellular Neuroscience 174*,10.

Hinton, V.J., Cyrulnik, S.E., Fee, R.J. *et al.* (2009) 'Association of autistic spectrum disorders with dystrophinopathies.' *Pediatric Neurology 41*, 5, 339–346.

Hinton, V.J., De Vivo, D.C., Nereo, N.E., Goldstein, E. and Stern, Y. (2000) 'Poor verbal working memory across intellectual level in boys with Duchenne dystrophy.' *Neurology 54*, 11, 2127–2132.

Hinton, V.J., De Vivo, D.C., Nereo, N.E., Goldstein, E. and Stern, Y. (2001) 'Selective deficits in verbal working memory associated with a known genetic etiology: The neuropsychological profile of duchenne muscular dystrophy.' *Journal of the International Neuropsychological Society: JINS 7*, 1, 45–54.

Humbertclaude, V., Hamroun, D., Picot, M.C. *et al.* (2013) 'Phenotypic heterogeneity and phenotype-genotype correlations in dystrophinopathies: Contribution of genetic and clinical databases.' *Revue Neurologique (Paris) 169*, 8–9, 583–594.

Kaplan, B.J., Dewey, D.M., Crawford, S.G. and Wilson, B.N. (2001) 'The term comorbidity is of questionable value in reference to developmental disorders: Data and theory.' *Journal of Learning Disabilities 34*, 6, 555–565.

LeDoux, J. (2003) 'The emotional brain, fear, and the amygdala.' *Cellular and Molecular Neurobiology 23*, 4–5, 727–738.

Lee, J.S., Pfund, Z., Juhasz, C. *et al.* (2002) 'Altered regional brain glucose metabolism in Duchenne muscular dystrophy: A pet study.' *Muscle and Nerve 26*, 4, 506–512.

Lidov, H.G. (1996) 'Dystrophin in the nervous system.' *Brain Pathology 6*, 1, 63–77.

Lorusso, M.L., Civati, F., Molteni, M., Turconi, A.C., Bresolin, N. and D'Angelo, M.G. (2013) 'Specific profiles of neurocognitive and reading functions in a sample of 42 Italian boys with Duchenne Muscular Dystrophy.' *Child Neuropsychology 19*, 4, 350–369.

Maresh, K.E., Muntoni, F (2017). *Deep phenotyping of the central nervous system in dystrophinopathies [Poster].* 10th UK Neuromuscular Translational Research Conference, London, March 2017.

McDonald, A.J. and Mott, D.D. (2017) 'Functional neuroanatomy of amygdalohippocampal interconnections and their role in learning and memory.' *Journal Neuroscience Research 95*, 3, 797–820.

McKenzie, K., Milton, M., Smith, G. and Ouellette-Kuntz, H. (2016) 'Systematic review of the prevalence and incidence of intellectual disabilities: Current trends and issues.' *Current Developmental Disorders Reports 3*, 2, 104–115.

Muntoni, F., Torelli, S. and Ferlini, A. (2003) 'Dystrophin and mutations: One gene, several proteins, multiple phenotypes.' *The Lancet Neurology 2*, 12, 731–740.

NHS Health Education England Genomics Education Programme Image Library (2014) Available at www.genomicseducation.hee.nhs.uk/resources, accessed on 07 December 2016.

Nico, B., Roncali, L., Mangieri, D. and Ribatti, D. (2005) 'Blood-brain barrier alterations in MDX mouse, an animal model of the Duchenne muscular dystrophy.' *Current Neurovascular Research 2*, 1, 47–54.

Niks, E.H. and Aartsma-Rus, A. (2017) 'Exon skipping: A first in class strategy for Duchenne muscular dystrophy.' *Expert Opinion on Biological Therapy 17*, 2, 225–236.

OpenStax CNX (2015) 'Psychology Collection: The Biology of Emotions.' Available at www.quizover.com/course/section/amygdala-emotion-by-openstax, accessed on 10 July 2017.

OpenStax, Anatomy & Physiology. *Chapter 26.1 Body Fluids and Compartments.* OpenStax CNX. Feb 26, 2016. http://cnx.org/contents/14fb4ad7-39a1-4eee-ab6e-3ef2482e3e22@8.24, accessed 10 July 2017.

Pane, M., Lombardo, M.E., Alfieri, P. *et al.* (2012) 'Attention deficit hyperactivity disorder and cognitive function in Duchenne muscular dystrophy: Phenotype-genotype correlation.' *The Journal of Pediatrics 161*, 4, 705–709.

Pane, M., Messina, S., Bruno, C. *et al.* (2013) 'Duchenne muscular dystrophy and epilepsy.' *Neuromuscular Disorders: NMD 23*, 4, 313–315.

Parsons, E.P., Clarke, A.J. and Bradley, D.M. (2004) 'Developmental progress in Duchenne muscular dystrophy: Lessons for earlier detection.' *European Journal of Paediatric Neurology 8*, 3, 145–153.

Perronnet, C. and Vaillend, C. (2010) 'Dystrophins, utrophins, and associated scaffolding complexes: Role in mammalian brain and implications for therapeutic strategies.' *Journal of Biomedicine and Biotechnology 2010*, 849426.

Ricotti, V., Jagle, H., Theodorou, M., Moore, A.T., Muntoni, F. and Thompson, D.A. (2016a) 'Ocular and neurodevelopmental features of Duchenne muscular dystrophy: A signature of dystrophin function in the central nervous system.' *European Journal of Human Genetics: EJHG 24*, 4, 562–568.

Ricotti, V., Mandy, W.P., Scoto, M. *et al.* (2016b) 'Neurodevelopmental, emotional, and behavioural problems in Duchenne muscular dystrophy in relation to underlying dystrophin gene mutations.' *Developmental Medicine and Child Neurology 58*, 1, 77–84.

Sekiguchi, M., Zushida, K., Yoshida, M. *et al.* (2009) 'A deficit of brain dystrophin impairs specific amygdala GABAergic transmission and enhances defensive behaviour in mice.' *Brain: A Journal of Neurology 132*, Pt 1, 124–135.

Smith, R.A., Sibert, J.R., Wallace, S.J. and Harper, P.S. (1989) 'Early diagnosis and secondary prevention of Duchenne muscular dystrophy.' *Archives of Disease in Childhood 64*, 6, 787–790.

Snow, W.M., Anderson, J.E. and Jakobson, L.S. (2013) 'Neuropsychological and neurobehavioral functioning in Duchenne muscular dystrophy: A review.' *Neuroscience and Biobehavioral Reviews 37*, 5, 743–752.

Suzuki, Y., Higuchi, S., Aida, I., Nakajima, T. and Nakada, T. (2017) 'Abnormal distribution of $GABA_A$ receptors in brain of Duchenne Muscular Dystrophy patients.' *Muscle and Nerve 2017 55*, 4, 591–595.

Taylor, P.J., Betts, G.A., Maroulis. S. *et al.* (2010) 'Dystrophin gene mutation location and the risk of cognitive impairment in Duchenne muscular dystrophy.' *PloS one 5,* 1, e8803.

Vacca, O., Charles-Messance, H., El Mathari, B. *et al.* (2016) 'AAV-mediated gene therapy in Dystrophin-Dp71 deficient mouse leads to blood-retinal barrier restoration and oedema reabsorption.' *Human Molecular Genetics 25,* 14, 3070–3079.

Vaillend, C., Perronnet, C., Ros, C. *et al.* (2010) 'Rescue of a dystrophin-like protein by exon skipping in vivo restores GABAA-receptor clustering in the hippocampus of the mdx mouse.' *Molecular Therapy: The Journal of the American Society of Gene Therapy 18,* 9, 1683–1688.

Van Naarden Braun, K., Christensen, D., Doernberg, N. *et al.* (2015) 'Trends in the prevalence of autism spectrum disorder, cerebral palsy, hearing loss, intellectual disability, and vision impairment, metropolitan atlanta, 1991–2010.' *PloS one 10,* 4, e0124120.

Waite, A., Brown, S.C. and Blake, D.J. (2012) 'The dystrophin–glycoprotein complex in brain development and disease.' *Trends in Neurosciences 35,* 8, 487–496.

Wu, J.Y., Kuban, K.C., Allred, E., Shapiro, F. and Darras, B.T. (2005) 'Association of Duchenne muscular dystrophy with autism spectrum disorder.' *Journal of Child Neurology 20,* 10, 790–795.

Xu, S., Shi, D., Pratt, S.J., Zhu, W., Marshall, A. and Lovering, R.M. (2015) 'Abnormalities in brain structure and biochemistry associated with mdx mice measured by in vivo MRI and high resolution localized (1)H MRS.' *Neuromuscular Disorders 25,* 10, 764–772.

Chapter 2

Anderson, S.W. Routh, D.K. and Ionasescu, V.V. (1988) 'Serial position memory of boys with Duchenne muscular dystrophy.' *Developmental Medicine and Child Neurology 30,* 3, 328–333.

Astrea, G., Pecini, C., Gasperini, F. *et al.* (2015) 'Reading impairment in Duchenne muscular dystrophy: A pilot study to investigate similarities and differences with developmental dyslexia.' *Research in Developmental Disabilities 45–46,* 168–177.

Banihani, R., Smile, S., Yoon, G., Dupuis, A., Mosleh, M., Snider, A. and McAdam, L. (2015) 'Cognitive and neurobehavioral profile in boys with Duchenne Muscular Dystrophy.' *Journal of Child Neurology 30,* 11, 1472–1482. *Developmental Medicine and Child Neurology 40,* 1, 12–20.

Billard, C., Gillet, P., Signoret, J.L. *et al.* (1992) 'Cognitive functions in Duchenne muscular dystrophy: A reappraisal and comparison with spinal muscular atrophy.' *Neuromuscular Disorders 2,* 5–6, 371–378.

Bresolin, N., Castelli, E., Comi, G.P. *et al.* (1994) 'Cognitive impairment in Duchenne muscular dystrophy.' *Neuromuscular Disorders 4*, 4, 359–369.

Bushby, K., Finkel, R., Birnkrant, D.J. *et al.* (2010) 'Diagnosis and management of Duchenne muscular dystrophy, part 1: Diagnosis, and pharmacological and psychosocial management.' *The Lancet Neurology 9*, 1, 77–93.

Bushby, K., Raybould, S., O'Donnell, S. and Steele, J.G. (2001) 'Social deprivation in Duchenne muscular dystrophy: Population based study.' *British Medical Journal 323*, 7320, 1035–1036.

Chen, J.-Y. (2008) 'Mediators affecting family function in families of children with Duchenne Muscular Dystrophy.' *The Kaohsiung Journal of Medical Sciences 24*, 10, 514–522.

Chen, J.-Y. and Clark, M.-J. (2007) 'Family function in families of children with Duchenne muscular dystrophy.' *Family and Community Health 30*, 4, 296–304.

Chen, J.-Y. and Clark, M.-J. (2010) 'Family resources and parental health in families of children with Duchenne Muscular Dystrophy. *Journal of Nursing Research 18*, 4, 239–248.

Chieffo, D., Brogna, C., Berardinelli, A. *et al.* (2015) 'Early neurodevelopmental findings predict school age cognitive abilities in Duchenne Muscular Dystrophy: A longitudinal study.' *PLoS One 10*, 8, e0133214.

Condly, S.J. (2006) 'Resilience in children: A review of literature with implications for education.' *Urban Education 41*, 3, 211–236.

Connolly, A.M., Florence, J.M., Cradock, M.M. *et al.* (2013) 'Motor and cognitive assessment of infants and young boys with Duchenne Muscular Dystrophy: Results from the Muscular Dystrophy Association DMD Clinical Research Network.' *Neuromuscular Disorders 23*, 7, 529–539.

Connolly, A.M., Florence, J.M., Cradock, M.M. *et al.* (2014) 'One year outcome of boys with Duchenne muscular dystrophy using the Bayley-III scales of infant and toddler development.' *Pediatric Neurology 50*, 6, 557–563.

Cotton, S., Crowe, S.F. and Voudouris, N. (1998) 'Neuropsychological profile of Duchenne muscular dystrophy.' *Child Neuropsychology 4*, 110–117.

Cotton, S., Voudouris, N.J. and Greenwood, K.M. (2001) 'Intelligence and Duchenne muscular dystrophy: Full-scale, verbal, and performance intelligence quotients.' *Developmental Medicine and Child Neurology 43*, 7, 497–501.

Cotton, S.M., Voudouris, N.J. and Greenwood, K.M. (2005) 'Association between intellectual functioning and age in children and young adults with Duchenne muscular dystrophy: Further results from a meta-analysis.' *Developmental Medicine and Child Neurology 47*, 4, 257–265.

Cyrulnik, S.E., Fee, R.J., Batchelder, A., Kiefel, J., Goldstein, E. and Hinton, V.J. (2008) 'Cognitive and adaptive deficits in young children with Duchenne muscular dystrophy (DMD).' *Journal of the International Neuropsychological Society 14*, 5, 853–861.

Darke, J., Bushby, K., Le Couteur, A. and McConachie, H. (2006) 'Survey of behaviour problems in children with neuromuscular diseases.' *European Journal of Paediatric Neurology 10*, 3, 129–134.

Donders, J. and Taneja, C. (2009) 'Neurobehavioral characteristics of children with Duchenne Muscular Dystrophy.' *Child Neuropsychology 15*, 3, 295–304.

Elsenbruch, S., Schmid, J., Lutz, S., Geers, B. and Schara, U. (2013) 'Self-reported quality of life and depressive symptoms in children, adolescents, and adults with duchenne muscular dystrophy: A cross-sectional survey study.' *Neuropediatrics 44*, 5, 257–264.

Engel de Abreu, P.M. and Gathercole, S.E. (2012) 'Executive and phonological processes in second-language acquisition.' *Journal of Educational Psychology 104*, 4, 974.

Fabbro, F., Marini, A., Felisari, G., Comi, G.P., D'Angelo, M.G., Turconi, A.C. and Bresolin, N. (2007) 'Language disturbances in a group of participants suffering from Duchenne muscular dystrophy: A pilot study.' *Perceptual and Motor Skills 104*, 2, 663–676.

Fee, R.J. and Hinton, V.J. (2011) 'Resilience in children diagnosed with a chronic neuromuscular disorder.' *Journal of Developmental and Behavioral Pediatrics 32*, 9, 644–650.

Galuschka, K., Ise, E., Krick, K. and Schulte-Körne, G. (2014) 'Effectiveness of treatment approaches for children and adolescents with reading disabilities: A meta-analysis of randomized controlled trials.' *PLoS One 9*, 2, e89900.

Gathercole, S.E., Alloway, T.P., Willis, C. and Adams, A.-M. (2006) 'Working memory in children with reading disabilities.' *Journal of Experimental Child Psychology 93*, 3, 265–281.

Hendriksen, J.G. and Vles, J.S. (2006) 'Are males with Duchenne muscular dystrophy at risk for reading disabilities?' *Pediatric Neurology 34*, 4, 296–300.

Hendriksen, J.G. and Vles, J.S. (2008) 'Neuropsychiatric disorders in males with duchenne muscular dystrophy: Frequency rate of attention-deficit hyperactivity disorder (ADHD), autism spectrum disorder, and obsessive-compulsive disorder.' *Journal of Child Neurology 23*, 5, 477–481.

Hinton, V.J., Cyrulnik, S.E., Fee, R.J. *et al.* (2009) 'Association of autistic spectrum disorders with dystrophinopathies.' *Pediatric Neurology 41*, 5, 339–346.

Hinton, V.J., De Vivo, D.C., Nereo, N.E., Goldstein, E. and Stern, Y. (2000) 'Poor verbal working memory across intellectual level in boys with Duchenne dystrophy.' *Neurology 54*, 11, 2127–2132.

Hinton, V.J., De Vivo, D.C., Nereo, N.E., Goldstein, E. and Stern, Y. (2001) 'Selective deficits in verbal working memory associated with a known genetic etiology: The neuropsychological profile of duchenne muscular dystrophy.' *Journal of the International Neuropsychological Society 7*, 1, 45–54.

Hinton, V.J., DeVivo, D.C., Fee, R.J., Goldstein, E. and Stern, Y. (2004) 'Investigation of poor academic achievement in children with Duchenne muscular dystrophy.' *Learning Disabilites Research and Practice 19*, 146–154.

Hinton, V.J., Fee, R., Goldstein, E.M. and De Vivo, D.C. (2007a) 'Verbal and memory skills in males with Duchenne muscular dystrophy.' *Developmental Medicine and Child Neurology 49*, 2, 123–128.

Hinton, V.J., Fee, R.J., De Vivo, D.C. and Goldstein, E. (2007b) 'Poor facial affect recognition among boys with duchenne muscular dystrophy.' *Journal of Autism and Developmental Disorders 37*, 10, 1925–1933.

Hinton, V.J., Kim, S.Y., Fee, R.J., Goldstein, E. and DeVivo, D.C. (2016) 'Cognitive and behavioral gains over time in Duchenne muscular dystrophy.' *Unpublished manuscript.*

Hoskin, J. and Fawcett, A. (2014) 'Improving the reading skills of young people with Duchenne muscular dystrophy in preparation for adulthood.' *British Journal of Special Education 41*, 2, 172–190.

Karagan, N.J., Richman, L.C. and Sorensen, J.P. (1980) 'Analysis of verbal disability in Duchenne muscular dystrophy.' *Journal of Nervous and Mental Disease 168*, 7, 419–423.

Leaffer, E.B., Fee, R.J. and Hinton, V.J. (2016) 'Digit span performance in children with dystrophinopathy: A verbal span or working memory contribution?' *Journal of the International Neuropsychological Society: JINS*, 1–8.

Marini, A., Lorusso, M.L., D'Angelo, M.G., Civati, F., Turconi, A.C., Fabbro, F. and Bresolin, N. (2007) 'Evaluation of narrative abilities in patients suffering from Duchenne Muscular Dystrophy.' *Brain and Language 102*, 1, 1–12.

Mento, G., Tarantino, V. and Bisiacchi, P.S. (2011) 'The neuropsychological profile of infantile Duchenne muscular dystrophy.' *Clinical Neuropsychology 25*, 8, 1359–1377.

Nereo, N.E., Fee, R.J. and Hinton, V.J. (2003) 'Parental stress in mothers of boys with duchenne muscular dystrophy.' *Journal of Pediatric Psychology 28*, 7, 473–484.

Ogasawara, A. (1989) 'Downward shift in IQ in persons with Duchenne muscular dystrophy compared to those with spinal muscular atrophy.' *American Journal of Mental Retardation 93*, 5, 544–547.

Pane, M., Lombardo, M.E., Alfieri, P. *et al.* (2012) 'Attention deficit hyperactivity disorder and cognitive function in Duchenne muscular dystrophy: Phenotype-genotype correlation.' *Journal of Pediatrics 161*, 4, 705–709, e701.

Pane, M., Scalise, R., Berardinelli, A. *et al.* (2013) 'Early neurodevelopmental assessment in Duchenne muscular dystrophy.' *Neuromuscular Disorders 23*, 6, 451–455.

Poysky, J. (2007) 'Behavior patterns in Duchenne muscular dystrophy: Report on the Parent Project Muscular Dystrophy behavior workshop 8–9 of December 2006, Philadelphia, USA. *Neuromuscular Disorders 17*, 11–12, 986–994.

Rahbek, J., Werge, B., Madsen, A., Marquardt, J., Steffensen, B.F. and Jeppesen, J. (2005) 'Adult life with Duchenne muscular dystrophy: Observations among an emerging and unforeseen patient population.' *Pediatric Rehabilitation 8*, 1, 17–28.

Snow, W.M., Anderson, J.E. and Jakobson, L.S. (2013) 'Neuropsychological and neurobehavioral functioning in Duchenne muscular dystrophy: A review.' *Neuroscience and Biobehavioral Reviews 37*, 5, 743–752.

Sollee, N.D., Latham, E.E., Kindlon, D.J. and Bresnan, M.J. (1985) 'Neuropsychological impairment in Duchenne muscular dystrophy.' *Journal of Clinical and Experimental Neuropsychology 7*, 5, 486–496.

Steele, M., Taylor, E., Young, C., McGrath, P., Lyttle, B.D.B. and Davidson, B. (2008) 'Mental health of children and adolescents with Duchenne muscular dystrophy.' *Developmental Medicine and Child Neurology 50*, 8, 638–639.

Whelan, T.B. (1987) 'Neuropsychological performance of children with Duchenne muscular dystrophy and spinal muscle atrophy.' *Developmental Medicine and Child Neurology 29*, 2, 212–220.

Wicksell, R.K., Kihlgren, M., Melin, L. and Eeg-Olofsson, O. (2004) 'Specific cognitive deficits are common in children with Duchenne muscular dystrophy.' *Developmental Medicine and Child Neurology 46*, 3, 154–159.

Wu, J.Y., Kuban, K.C., Allred, E., Shapiro, F. and Darras, B.T. (2005) 'Association of Duchenne muscular dystrophy with autism spectrum disorder.' *Journal of Child Neurology 20*, 10, 790–795.

Chapter 3

Archer, J.E., Gardner, A.C., Roper, H.P., Chikermane, A.A. and Tatman, A.J. (2016) 'Duchenne muscular dystrophy: The management of scoliosis.' *Journal of Spine Surgery 2*, 185–194.

Emery, A. and Muntoni, F. (eds) (2003) *Duchenne Muscular Dystrophy* (3rd edition). Oxford: Oxford University Press.

Equality Act (2010) *Education Rights*. Available at www.gov.uk/rights-disabled-person/education-rights, accessed on 23 May 2017.

Fujiwara, T., Tanabe, A., Uchikawa, K., Tsuji, T., Tanuma, A., Hase, K. and Liu, M. (2009) 'Activities of daily living (ADL) structure of patients with Duchenne muscular dystrophy, including adults.' *Keio Journal of Medicine 58*, 223–226.

Henricson, E.K., Abresch, R.T., Cnaan, A. *et al.* (2013) 'The cooperative international neuromuscular research group Duchenne natural history study: Glucocorticoid treatment preserves clinically meaningful functional milestones and reduces rate of disease progression as measured by manual muscle testing and other: CINRG DMD Natural History Study.' *Muscle Nerve 48*, 55–67.

Honório, S., Batista, M. and Martins, J. (2013) 'The influence of hydrotherapy on obesity prevention in individuals with Duchenne Muscular Dystrophy.' *Journal of Physical Education and Sport 13*, 140.

Jansen, M., de Groot, I.J., van Alfen, N. and Geurts, A.C. (2010) 'Physical training in boys with Duchenne Muscular Dystrophy: The protocol of the No Use is Disuse study.' *BMC Pediatrics 10*, 55.

Katz, K., Rosenthal, A. and Yosipovitch, Z. (1992) 'Normal ranges of popliteal angle in children.' *Journal of Pediatric Orthopaedics 12*, 2, 229–231.

Larson, C.M and Henderson, R.C. (2000) 'Bone mineral density and fractures in boys with Duchenne Muscular Dystrophy.' *Journal of Pediatric Orthopaedics 20*, 1, 71.

Otto, C., Steffensen, B.F., Højberg, A.-L. *et al.* (2017) 'Predictors of Health-Related Quality of Life in boys with Duchenne muscular dystrophy from six European countries.' *Journal of Neurology 264*, 709–723.

Pane, M., Mazzone, E.S., Fanelli, L. *et al.* (2014) 'Reliability of the Performance of Upper Limb assessment in Duchenne muscular dystrophy.' *Neuromuscular Disorders 24*, 201–206.

Quinlivan, R., Roper, H., Davie, M., Shaw, N.J., McDonagh, J. and Bushby, K. (2005) 'Report of a Muscular Dystrophy Campaign funded workshop. Birmingham, UK, January 16th 2004. Osteoporosis in Duchenne muscular dystrophy; its prevalence, treatment and prevention.' *Neuromuscular Disorders 15*, 72–79.

Skalsky, A.J. and McDonald, C.M. (2012) 'Prevention and management of limb contractures in neuromuscular diseases.' *Physical Medicine and Rehabilitation Clinics of North America 23*, 675–687.

Useful links

NICE Guidelines for Ataluren (2016) www.nice.org.uk/guidance/hst3

www.treat-nmd.eu/resources/care-overview/dmd-care/dmd-care-standards-about

www.treat-nmd.eu/care/dmd/diagnosis-management-DMD

hwww.musculardystrophyuk.org

Chapter 4

Alexander-Passe, N. (2006) 'How dyslexic teenagers cope: An investigation of self-esteem, coping and depression'. *Dyslexia 12*, 256–275.

Alloway, T. and Alloway, R. (2010) 'Investigating the predictive roles of working memory and IQ in academic attainment.' *Journal of Experimental and Child Psychology 106*, 1, 20–29.

Astrea, G., Pecini, C., Gasperini, F. *et al.* (2015) 'Reading impairment in Duchenne muscular dystrophy: A pilot study to investigate similarities and differences with developmental dyslexia.' *Research in Developmental Disabilities 45–46,* 168–177.

Billard, C., Gillet, P., Barthez, M., Hommet, C. and Bertrand, P. (1998) 'Reading ability and processing in Duchenne muscular dystrophy and spinal muscular atrophy.' *Developmental Medicine and Child Neurology 40,* 1, 12–20.

Bishop, D.V.M. and Adams, C. (1990) 'A prospective study of the relationship between specific language impairment, phonological disorders and reading retardation.' *Journal of Child Psychology and Psychiatry* 31, 1027–1050.

Blatchford, P., Bassett, P., Brown, P., Martin, C., Russell, A., Webster, R. and Haywood, N. (2009) *The Deployment and Impact of Support Staff in Schools. Report on the Findings from Strand 1, Wave 1.* Department for Education and Skills (DfES). Research Report 776. Available at www.dcsf.gov.uk/research/data/uplo adfiles/RR776.pdf, accessed on 11 July 2017.

Bosanquet, P., Radford, J. and Webster, R. (2016) *The Teaching Assistant's Guide to Effective Interaction: How to Maximise Your Practice.* London: Routledge.

Bradley, L. and Bryant, P.E. (1983) 'Categorising sounds and learning to read: A causal connection.' *Nature 301,* 419–421

Brooks, G. and National Foundation for Educational Research (2007) *What Works for Children with Literacy Difficulties,* 3rd edition. London: DCSF.

Bushby, K., Finkel, R., Birnkrant, D.J. *et al.* (2010) 'DMD Care Considerations Working Group. Diagnosis and management of Duchenne Muscular dystrophy, Part 1: Diagnosis, and pharmacological and psychosocial management.' *Lancet Neurology 9,* 1.

Cotton, S., Voudouris, N.J. and Greenwood, K.M. (2001) 'Intelligence and Duchenne muscular dystrophy: Full-scale, verbal, and performance intelligence quotients.' *Developmental Medicine and Child Neurology 43,* 7, 497–501.

Cotton, S.M., Voudouris, N.J., and Greenwood, K.M. (2005) 'Association between intellectual functioning and age in children with Duchenne muscular dystrophy: Further results from a meta-analysis.' *Developmental Medicine and Child Neurology,* 47, 257–265.

Cyrulnik, S.E., Fee, R.J., De Vivo, D.C., Goldstein, E. and Hinton, V.J. (2007) 'Delayed developmental language milestones in children with Duchenne's muscular dystrophy.' *The Journal of Pediatrics 150,* 5, 474–478.

De Shazer, S. and Dolan, Y. (2007) *More than Miracles: The State of the Art of Solution-Focused Brief Therapy.* Abingdon: Haworth Press.

Ehri, L.C. (1995) 'Phases of development in learning to read by sight.' *Journal of Research in Reading 18,* 116–125

Ericsson, A. and Pool, R. (2017) *Peak – How All of Us Can Achieve Extraordinary Things,* 1st edition. New York: Vintage.

Frederickson, F. and Turner, J. (2003) 'Utilizing the classroom peer group to address children's social needs: An evaluation.' *The Journal of Special Education 36*, 4, 234.

Frith, U. (1999) 'The paradoxes in the definition of dyslexia.' *Dyslexia 5*, 4, 192–214.

Giangreco, M.F. (2010) 'One-to–one paraprofessionals for students with disabilities in inclusive classrooms: Is conventional wisdom wrong?' *Intellectual Developmental Disabilities 48*, 1–13

Green, R.W. (2014) *Lost at School: Why our Kids with Behavioural Challenges Are Falling through the Cracks and How We Can Help Them.* New York: Scribner.

Gough, P.B. and Tunmer, W.E. (1986) 'Decoding, reading and reading disability.' *Remedial and Special Education 7*, 6–10.

Gould, S.J. (1981) *The Mismeasure of Man.* New York: W.W. Norton and Company.

Hendriksen, J.G. and Vles, J.S. (2006) 'Are males with Duchenne muscular dystrophy at risk for reading disabilities?' *Pediatric Neurology 34.* 296–300.

Hinton, V.J., De Vivo, D.C., Nereo, N.E., Goldstein, E. and Stern, Y. (2000) 'Poor verbal working memory across intellectual level in boys with Duchenne dystrophy.' *Neurology 54*, 11, 2127–2132.

Hinton, V.J., Fee, R., Goldstein, E.M. and De Vivo, D.C. (2007) 'Verbal and memory skills in males with Duchenne muscular dystrophy.' *Developmental Medicine and Child Neurology 49*, 2, 123–128.

Hoskin, J. and Fawcett, A. (2014) 'Improving the reading skills of young people with Duchenne muscular dystrophy in preparation for adulthood.' *British Journal of Special Education 41*, 2, 172–190.

Kamin, L.J. (1977) *The Science and Politics of IQ.* Hammondsworth: Penguin.

Kaplan, L.C., Osborne, P. and Elias, E. (1986) 'The diagnosis of muscular dystrophy in patients referred for language delay.' *Journal of Child Psychology and Psychiatry 27*, 545–549.

Minow, M. (1985) 'Learning to live with the dilemma of difference: Bilingual and special education.' 48 *Law and Contemporary Problems* 157–211.

Nicolson, R.I., Fawcett A. and Dean, P. (2001) 'Developmental Dyslexia: The cerebellar deficit hypothesis.' *Trends in Neuroscience 30*, 4.

Rahbek, J., Werge, B., Madsen, A., Marquardt, J., Steffensen, B.F. and Jeppesen, J. (2005) 'Adult life with Duchenne muscular dystrophy: Observations among an emerging and unforeseen patient population.' *Pediatric Rehabilitation 8*, 1, 17–28.

Reid, G. (2016) *Dyslexia: A Practioner's Handbook,* 5th edition. London: Sage.

Rose, J. (2009) Identifying and teaching children and young people with dyslexia and literacy difficulties: An independent report from Sir Jim Rose to the Secretary of State for Children, Schools and Families. London: Department of Schools, Children and Families.

Smidt, S. (2011) *Playing to Learn: The Role of Play in the Early Years.* Abingdon: Routledge.

Smith, R.A., Sibert, J.R., Wallace, S.J. and Harper, P.S. (1989) 'Early diagnosis and secondary prevention of Duchenne muscular dystrophy.' *Archives of Disabled Children 64*, 6, 787–790.

Snowling, M. (2000) *Dyslexia*. Oxford: Basil Blackwell

Stanovich, K.E.(1986) 'Matthew effects in reading: Some consequences of individual differences in the acquisition of literacy.' *Reading Research Quarterly 21*, 4, 360.

Stanovich, K.E., (1996) 'Towards a more inclusive definition of Dyslexia.' *Dyslexia 2* 154–166.

Torgeson, J.K. (2006) Recent Discoveries on Remedial Interventions for Children with Dyslexia.' In Snowling, M. and Hulme, C. (eds) *The Science of Reading: A Handbook*. Oxford: Blackwell Publishers.

The Royal Society (2011) Brainwaves Module II Neuroscience: Implications for Education and Life long Learning RS Policy document 02/11 Issued: February 2011 DES2105.

Vellutino, F.R., Fletcher, J.M., Snowling, M.J. and Scanlon, D.M (2004) 'Specific reading disability (dyslexia): What have we learned in the past four decades?' *Journal of Child Psychology and Psychiatry 45*, 1, 2–40.

Vygotsky, L.S. (1978) *Mind in Society: The Development of Higher Psychological Processes*. London: Harvard University Press.

Webster, R. and Blatchford, P. (2013) Worlds Apart? How pupils with statements lead a life away from the class. Findings from the Making a Statement Project Assessment and Development Matters, 5 (1), Leicester: British Psychological Society. Available online at www.maximisingtas.co.uk/research/the-mast-study.php, accessed on 11 July 2017.

Whelan, T.B. (1987) 'Neuropsychological performance of children with Duchenne muscular dystrophy and spinal muscle atrophy.' *Developmental Medicine and Child Neurology 29*, 2, 212–220.

Wolf, M. and Bowers, P.G. (1999) 'The double-deficit hypothesis for the developmental dyslexias.' *Journal of Educational Psychology 91*, 3, 415–438.

Woollett, K., Spiers, H.J. and Maguire, E.A. (2009) 'Talent in the taxi: A model system for exploring expertise.' *Philosophical Transactions of the Royal Society of B 364*, 1522, 1407–1416.

Worden, D.K. and Vignos, P.J. (1962) 'Intellectual function in childhood progressive muscular dystrophy.' *Pediatrics 29*, 968–977.

Chapter 5

Banihani, R., Smile, S., Yoon, G. *et al.* (2015) 'Cognitive and neurobehavioral profile in boys with Duchenne muscular dystrophy.' *Journal of Child Neurology 30*, 11, 1472–1482.

Cotton, S., Crowe, S.F. and Voudouris, N. (1998) 'Neuropsychological profile of Duchenne muscular dystrophy.' *Child Neuropsychology 4*, 2, 110–117.

Donders, J. and Taneja, C. (2009) 'Neurobehavioral characteristics of children with Duchenne muscular dystrophy.' *Child Neuropsychology 15*, 3, 295–304.

Doorenweerd, N., Straathof, C.S., Dumas, E.M. *et al.* (2014) 'Reduced cerebral gray matter and altered white matter in boys with Duchenne muscular dystrophy.' *Annals of Neurology 76*, 3, 403–411.

Fitzpatrick, C., Barry, C. and Garvey, C. (1986) 'Psychiatric disorder among boys with Duchenne muscular dystrophy.' *Developmental Medicine and Child Neurology 28*, 5, 589–595.

The Gottman Institute (2017) *Raising Emotionally Intelligent Children.* The Gottman Institute. Available at www.gottman.com, accessed on 30 April 2017.

Hendriksen, J.G. and Vles, J.S. (2006) 'Are males with Duchenne muscular dystrophy at risk for reading disabilities?' *Pediatric Neurology 34*, 4, 296–300.

Hinton, V.J., De Vivo, D.C., Nereo, N.E. *et al.* (2000) 'Poor verbal working memory across intellectual level in boys with Duchenne dystrophy.' *Neurology 54*, 11, 2127–2132.

Hinton, V.J., Nereo, N.E., Fee, R.J. and Cyrulnik, S.E. (2006) 'Social behavior problems in boys with Duchenne muscular dystrophy. *Journal of Developmental and Behavioral Pediatrics 27*, 6, 470–476.

Lives in the Balance (2017) Available at www.livesinthebalance.org, accessed on 30 April 2017.

Nereo, N.E. and Hinton, V.J. (2003) 'Three wishes and psychological functioning in boys with Duchenne muscular dystrophy.' *Journal of Developmental and Behavioral Pediatrics 24*, 2, 96–103.

Nereo N.E., Fee R.J. and Hinton, V.J. (2003) 'Parental stress in mothers of boys with Duchenne muscular dystrophy'. *J Pediatr Psychol. 28*, 7, 473–484.

Perumal, A.R., Rajeswaran, J. and Nalini, A. (2015) 'Neuropsychological profile of Duchenne muscular dystrophy.' *Applied Neuropsychology: Child 4*, 1, 49–57.

Poysky, J. and Behavior in DMD Study Group (2007) 'Behavior patterns in Duchenne muscular dystrophy: Report on the Parent Project Muscular Dystrophy behavior workshop 8–9 of December 2006, Philadelphia, USA.' *Neuromuscular Disorders 17*, 11–12, 986–994.

Chapter 7

AandE App Duchenne Muscular Dystrophy (2015) *Introduction to A and E Care for Duchenne muscular dystrophy.* Available at www.duchenneemergency.co.uk, accessed on 17 October 2016.

Baddeley, A. (1992) 'Working memory.' *Science 255*, 5044, 556–559.

Brief.org.uk (2016) *BRIEF - The Centre for Solution Focused Practice.* Available at www.brief.org.uk, accessed on 16 November 2016.

Bushby, K., Finkel, R., Birnkrant, D. *et al.* (2010a) 'Diagnosis and management of Duchenne muscular dystrophy, part 1: Diagnosis, and pharmacological and psychosocial management.' Available at www.thelancet.com/journals/lancet/article/PIIS1474-4422(09)70271-6/fulltext, accessed on 22 May 2017.

Bushby, K., Finkel, R., Birnkrant, D. *et al.* (2010b) 'Diagnosis and management of Duchenne muscular dystrophy, part 2: Implementation of multidisciplinary care.' Available at www.thelancet.com/journals/laneur/article/PIIS1474-4422(09)70272-8/fulltext, accessed 22 May 2017.

Children and Families Act (2014) Available at www.legislation.gov.uk/ukpga/2014/6/contents/enacted, accessed on 25 May 2017.

Chronically Sick and Disabled Persons Act (1970) Available at www.legislation.gov.uk/ukpga/1970/44/section/2, accessed on 25 May 2017.

Council for Disabled Children (2017) Education Health and Care Plans – Examples of Good Practice. Available at www.councilfordisabledchildren.org.uk/sites/default/files/field/attachemnt/EHCP%20Exemplar%20Guide%202017.pdf, accessed 15 March 2017.

Cyrulnik, S., Fee, R., De Vivo, D., Goldstein, E. and Hinton, V. (2007) 'Delayed developmental language milestones in children with Duchenne's Muscular Dystrophy.' *The Journal of Pediatrics 150*, 5, 474–478.

de Shazer, S. and Berg, I. (1997) '"What works?" Remarks on research aspects of Solution-Focused Brief Therapy.' *Journal of Family Therapy 19*, 2, 121–124.

Department for Education and Department of Health (2014) *Special Educational Needs and Disability Code of Practice: 0 to 25 years.* Available at www.gov.uk/government/uploads/system/uploads/attachment_data/file/398815/SEND_Code_of_Practice_January_2015.pdf, accessed on 11 October 2016.

Disabilityrightsuk.org. (2017) *Personal budgets helpline | Disability Rights UK.* Available at: www.disabilityrightsuk.org/how-we-can-help/helplines/independent-living-advice-line, accessed on 16 March 2017.

Ericsson, A. and Pool, R. (2017) *Peak – How All of Us Can Achieve Extraordinary Things* (1st edition), New York: Vintage.

Gathercole, S. and Packiam Alloway, T. (2007) *Understanding Working Memory - A Classroom Guide* (1st edition) [ebook]. Available at www.mrc-cbu.cam.ac.uk/wp-content/uploads/2013/01/WM-classroom-guide.pdf, accessed on 18 May 2017.

Gitsam, N. and Jordan, L. (2015) *The Preparing for Adulthood Review – A Good Practice Toolkit.* Available at www.preparingforadulthood.org.uk/media/385562/2upload.pfatoolkit.pdf, accessed on 6 October 2016.

Greene, R. (2017) *ALSUP.* Lives in the Balance. Available at www.livesinthebalance.org/sites/default/files/ALSUP216.pdf, accessed on 15 March 2017.

Hinton, V., De Vivo, D., Nereo, N., Goldstein, E. and Stern, Y. (2000) 'Poor verbal working memory across intellectual level in boys with Duchenne dystrophy.' *Neurology 54*, 11, 2127–2132.

Hinton, V., De Vivo, D., Nereo, N., Goldstein, E. and Stern, Y. (2001) 'Selective deficits in verbal working memory associated with a known genetic etiology: The neuropsychological profile of Duchenne muscular dystrophy.' *Journal of the International Neuropsychological Society 7*, 1, 45–54.

Hinton, V., Fee, R., Goldstein, E. and De Vivo, D. (2007) 'Verbal and memory skills in males with Duchenne muscular dystrophy.' *Developmental Medicine and Child Neurology 49*, 2, 123–128.

Hoskin, J. and Fawcett, A. (2014) 'Improving the reading skills of young people with Duchenne muscular dystrophy in preparation for adulthood.' *British Journal of Special Education 41*, 2, 172–190.

IPSEA (2014) *IPSEA Education Health and Care Plan Checklist.* Available at www.ipsea.org.uk/news/2014/education-health-and-care-plan-checklist, accessed 11 October 2016.

Jcq.org.uk (2017) *Access Arrangements and Reasonable Adjustments 2016–2017 – JCQ Joint Council for Qualifications.* Available at www.jcq.org.uk/exams-office/access-arrangements-and-special-consideration/regulations-and-guidance/access-arrangements-and-reasonable-adjustments-2016-2017, accessed on 22 May 2017.

Manual Handling HSE (2016) *Manual handling assessment charts (MAC) tool.* Available at www.hse.gov.uk/msd/mac, accessed on 17 October 2016.

Murray, M. (2009) *Safeguarding disabled children.* London: Department for Children, Schools and Families. Available at: www.gov.uk/government/uploads/system/uploads/attachment_data/file/190544/00374-2009DOM-EN.pdf, accessed on 17 October 2016.

Nhs.uk (2016) *NHS continuing healthcare – Care and support guide – NHS Choices.* Available at www.nhs.uk/Conditions/social-care-and-support-guide/Pages/nhs-continuing-care.aspx, accessed on 15 November 2016.

Poysky, J. (2011) *Learning and Behavior in Duchenne Muscular Dystrophy for parents and educators.* Available at www.parentprojectmd.org/site/DocServer/Learning_and_Behavior_Guide.pdf?docID=11001, accessed on 8 November 2016.

Preparingforadulthood.org.uk (2016) *Stories | Preparing for Adulthood.* Available at: www.preparingforadulthood.org.uk/resources/stories?page=1, accessed on 6 October 2016.

Preparing for Adulthood (2017) *PfA Outcomes Tool.* Available at www.preparingforadulthood.org.uk/media/442444/final_dfe_-_no_bullets_-_pfa_outcomes_tool.pdf, accessed on 15 March 2017.

Ricotti, V., Mandy, W., Scoto, M. *et al.* (2015) 'Neurodevelopmental, emotional, and behavioural problems in Duchenne muscular dystrophy in relation to underlying dystrophin gene mutations.' *Developmental Medicine and Child Neurology 58*, 1, 77–84.

Risk Assessments Hertfordshire Grid (2016) *HGfL: School Admin: School Office: Health and Safety: Risk Assessments.* Available at www.thegrid.org.uk/info/healthandsafety/risk_assessment.shtml, accessed on 17 October 2016.

Rix Centre UEL (2016) *RIX Media | RIX Research and Media.* Available at www.rixresearchandmedia.org/rix/home-media, accessed on 6 October 2016.

Sanderson, H. (2013) *Person-Centred Reviews film.* Available at www.youtube.com/watch?v=bkwBSF0nxiYandindex=1andlist=PLjB3u9kDbySHyfp6t 3BPWjZu2bsQrnFfc, accessed on 6 October 2016.

Treat-nmd.eu (2016) *TREAT-NMD: Family guide.* Available at www.treat-nmd.eu/care/dmd/family-guide, accessed on 5 October 2016.

Villanova, M. and Kazibwe, S. (2017) 'New survival target for Duchenne Muscular Dystrophy.' *American Journal of Physical Medicine and Rehabilitation 96*, 2, e28–e30.

Vry, J., Gramsch, K., Rodger, S. *et al.* (2016) 'European cross-sectional survey of current care practices for Duchenne Muscular Dystrophy reveals regional and age-dependent differences.' *Journal of Neuromuscular Diseases 3*, 4, 517–527.

Chapter 8

Abbott, D., Carpenter, J. and Bushby, K. (2012) 'Transition to adulthood for young men with Duchenne muscular dystrophy: Research from the UK.' *Neuromuscular Disorders 22*, 445–446.

Beresford, B. and Stuttard, L. (2014) 'Young adult users of adult healthcare: Experiences of young adults with complex or life-limiting conditions'. *Clinical Medicine, 14*, 4, 404–408.

Care Quality Commission (2014) *From the Pond Into the Sea Children's Transition to Adult Health Services.* Available at www.cqc.org.uk/sites/default/files/CQC_ Transition%20Report.pdf, accessed on 12 July 2017.

Decipha CIC (2014) Living with Duchenne Animation. Available at www.youtube.com/watch?v=mltKe5tyzk8andt=21s, accessed on 12 July 2017.

Department for Education (2014) Special Educational Needs and Disability Pathfinder Programme Evaluation Thematic Report: The Education, Health and Care (EHC) Planning Pathway for families that are new to the SEN system Research Report. Reference: DFE- RR326B.

Department for Education (2015) The Special Educational Needs and Disability Pathfinder Programme Evaluation Final Impact Research Report. Reference: DFE-RB471.

Department for Education and Department of Health (2015) *Special Educational Needs and Disability Code of Practice 0 to 25 Years>* Available at www.gov.uk/government/publications/send-code-of-praactice-0-to-25. Accessed on 2 June 2017.

Department for Education (2016) *Mapping User Experiences of the Education Health and Care Process: A Qualitative Study.* Reference: DFE-RR523.

Department of Health (2010) Valuing People Now Summary Report March 2009 – September 2010. Available at www.gov.uk/government/uploads/system/uploads/attachment_data/file/215892/dh_122388.pdf. Accessed on 20 December 2017.

Department for Work and Pensions (August 2016) part of: Pre-work Programme, New Enterprise Allowance and Employment Schemes statistics.

Eagle, M., Bourke, J., Bullock, R. *et al.* (2007) 'Managing Duchenne muscular dystrophy–the additive effect of spinal surgery and home nocturnal ventilation in improving survival.' *Neuromuscular Disorders 17*, 470–475.

Eakes, G.G., Burke, M.L. and Hainsworth, M.A. (1998) 'Middle-range theory of Chronic Sorrow.' *Journal of Nursing Scholarship 30*, 179–184.

Gibson, B.E., Mistry, B., Smith, B., Yoshida, K.K., Abbott, D., Lindsay, S. and Hamdani, Y. (2014) 'Becoming men: Gender, disability, and transitioning to adulthood.' *Health 18*, 1, 95–114.

Hoskin, J. (2017) 'Taking Charge and letting go: Exploring the ways a Transition to Adulthood project for teenagers with Duchenne Muscular Dystrophy has supported parents to prepare for the future'. *British Journal of Special Education 44*, 2, 165–185.

Kenwrick, S. (2016) 'Being a carrier for Duchenne Muscular Dystrophy.' Available at www.actionduchenne.org/dmd-carrier-leaflet, accessed on 12 July 2017.

Open University (2016) 'Talking about sex, sexuality and relationships: Guidance and standards for those working with young people with life-limiting or life-threatening conditions.' Available at www.open.ac.uk/health-and-social-care/research/sexuality-alliance, accessed on 12 July 2017.

Rahbek, J., Werge, B., Madsen, A., Fynbo, C. Steffensen, B. and Jeppesen, J. (2005) 'Adult life with Duchenne muscular dystrophy: Observations among an emerging and unforeseen patient population.' *Paediatric Rehabilitation 8*, 1, 17–28.

Runswick-Cole, K. and Goodley, D. (2013) 'Resilience: A disability studies and community psychology approach'. *Social and Personality Psychology Compass 7*, 67–78.

Sayce, L. (2011) 'Getting in, staying in and getting on: disability employment support for the future.' London: Department for Work and Pensions.

Schrans, D.G., Abbott, D., Peay, H.L. *et al.* (2013) 'Transition in Duchenne muscular dystrophy: An expert meeting report and description of transition needs in an emergent patient population: (parent project muscular dystrophy transition expert meeting 17–18 June 2011, Amsterdam, The Netherlands).' *Neuromuscular Disorders 23*, 3, 283–286.

Useful links

Preparing for Adulthood: www.preparingforadulthood.org

National Development Team for Inclusion: www.ndti.org.uk/uploads/files/ How_to_Support_Young_People_With_Special_Educational_Needs_into_ Work.pdf

Disability Confident: www.youtube.com/disabilityconfident

Getting a Life Pathways: www.gettingalife.org.uk

Aspirations for Life: www.aspirationsforlife.org

Case studies of young people on supported internships and information leaflet on EmployAbility at: www.preparingforadulthood.org.uk/delivering

Subject Index

Page numbers in *italics* refer to figures and tables.

Author Index